In Search
OF THE
Miraculous

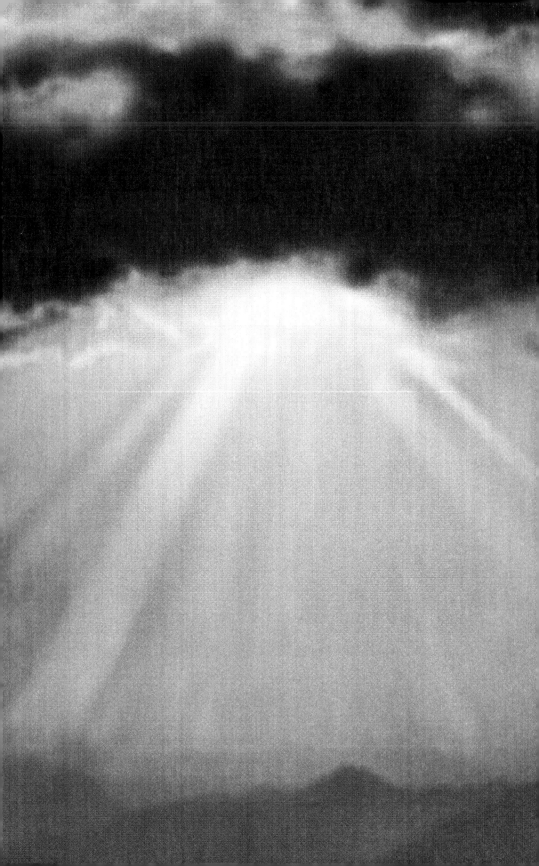

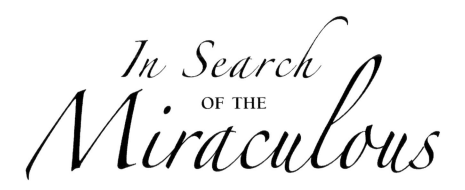

In Search
OF THE
Miraculous

A Guide to Overcoming

Addiction, Depression,

Eating Disorders, Heartbreak,

Obsession, Panic Attacks,

Phobias, and the Stronghold of

Compulsive Emotions,

such as Rage and Fear

EHSIDA BISSET

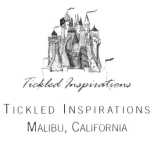

Tickled Inspirations

TICKLED INSPIRATIONS
MALIBU, CALIFORNIA

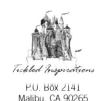

Tickled Inspirations
P.O. Box 2141
Malibu, CA 90265

The information contained in this book is intended to be educational and not for diagnostic, prescription, or treatment of any medical disorder whatsoever. The intent of the author is to offer information to help you in your quest for emotional and spiritual well-being. The content of this book is offered as an adjunct to a rational and responsible healthcare program prescribed by a healthcare practitioner. The author is in no way liable for any misuse of the material and assumes no responsibility for your actions.

In order to avoid sexism, the personal pronouns, "he and she" have been alternated through-out the book.

Publisher's Cataloging-in-Publication
(Provided by Quality Books, Inc.)

Bisset, Ehsida.
    In search of the miraculous : a guide to overcoming addiction, depression, eating disorders, heartbreak, obsession, panic attacks, phobias, and the stronghold of compulsive emotions, such as rage and fear / Ehsida Bisset. — 1st ed.
    p. cm.
    LCCN 2007907423
    ISBN-13: 978-0-9794843-0-8
    ISBN-10: 0-9794843-0-8

    1. Dependency (Psychology) 2. Personality.
3. Self-actualization (Psychology)   I. Title.

BF575.D34B57 2007   158.1
                      QBI07-600274

Printed in the U.S.A. First Edition August 2007

COMPILATION EDIT: Renee J. Wilson, Editor - Mentor
DEVELOPMENTAL/COPYEDIT: Carol Givner, Novelist – Editor
COVER AND INTERIOR DESIGN: Dotti Albertine
SHELL ART AND SEA LIFE DRAWING: Ehsida Bisset

Dedicated to

Existence

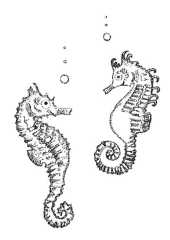

Special Thanks

To my extraordinary parents, who inspire me to live each moment with reverence. To Renee J. Wilson for her unfaltering patience, constant support, love, understanding, intelligence, generosity, and trust. To Michael Theodore for his boundless love, gentleness, benevolence, wisdom, and strength.

To Carol Givner for her brilliance, eloquence, integrity and kindness. And to all my magnificent clients who contributed their experiences to this book and continually choose a path which leads to higher levels of consciousness.

My gratitude is eternal and infinite.

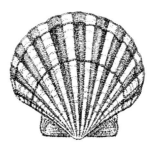

Acknowledgments

Every book is a compilation of influences the author has encountered. Although this manuscript arises from my own personal experience, many on my path have illuminated these realizations.

It would take an entire volume to acknowledge each person who stimulated these insights, but there are a few who contributed more significantly. Shirley MacLaine opened my eyes to Jane Roberts and the Seth Material, which inspired interest in the works of Albert Einstein, Nicola Tesla, Stephen Hawking, Johannes Kepler, Wilhelm Reich and Rudolf Steiner; which led to the insights of George Gurdjieff, P.D. Ouspensky, Krishnamurti, Patanjali, Lao Tzu, Masto and most significantly Pythagoras and Osho.

The brilliant compilations of Riso and Hudson, Louise L. Hay, David R. Hawkins M.D., Ph.D., Catherine Ponder, Abraham (Esther and Jerry Hicks) Gerber and A.A. Milne, all figured significantly in this manuscript. I would like to thank all these brilliant and wise beings for their profound insights into the human condition and their extraordinary ability to convey deep truths.

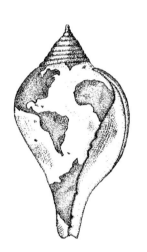

Contents

PART TWO

Case studies of people who have applied The Witnessing
Technique to rise above their painful programming

PART ONE

An Introduction to
"The Mind" and Pure Consciousness

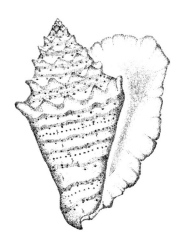

CHAPTER 1

In Search of the Miraculous

Introduction

SPOTTING A RAINBOW THROUGH A MIST, awakening to the first call of a songbird at dawn, or drinking in the scent of jasmine on a summer breeze; we wish these moments could last forever. A blooming rose, the lullaby of crickets, and the splashing of a waterfall all stir something sacred deep within. Nature ignites an intense longing, which we often have difficulty identifying. It is a longing to be filled with this same mysterious beauty.

These precious glimpses cannot last forever, but the euphoria they trigger can. Our yearning will not be quenched by consuming or possessing the beauty which attracts us. We must become one with the very essence we find intangible.

The further away from nature we go, the greater our desire for stimulants that keep us calm amid the sting of each day. We seek fulfillment from objects, subjects, behaviors, and substances in the physical world, which we hope will ease our pain and calm our fears forever. Yet, we are only left aching for more.

Dependence within society is a desperate race to escape our disappointment of the world and its inability to fulfill our soul. To move beyond addiction, anxiety, compulsions, depression, eating disorders, heartbreak, obsession, panic attacks, phobias, and neurosis of any kind, we must discover how to merge once again with the mystifying grace of Existence.

Neutrality

One source of energy flows through Existence. This power is the creative force which brings forth life and inspiration. It has been given many names, among them: Life Force, Universal Intelligence, Essence, Divinity, Liquid Light, Chi, Prana, Ki, Unconditional Love, Pure Consciousness, and Harmonia Macrocosmica.

Mystics and scientists agree that the energy itself is neutral and exists without persuasion, categorization, or limitation. Sunlight skipping across the ocean, moonbeams illuminating the night, and raindrops dancing in the sky all demonstrate neutrality. They share their blessings equally with the tiniest blade of grass to the tallest tree. Nature is a pure expression of the Divine.

Free Will

Plants, wild animals, and the elements all pulse with the neutral energy of Pure Consciousness. When this neutral energy is filtered through the human apparatus, a similar expression of beauty and grace is possible. Humans possess a quality, however, which plant, animal, and elemental life do not. Humans have *free will* to determine how they will orchestrate, express, and experience their neutral energy or Life Force.

Free will is accompanied by the human mind, which is the antithesis of neutrality. The mind's perceptions are formed around categorizations, judgments, boundaries, limitations, calculations, conflict, and completions. Thus, the mind cannot align with the neutral, non-judgmental, boundless, unlimited, infinite, symbiotic, timeless, synchronicity of Pure Consciousness.

Because the mind is formed by *duality*, (right and wrong, good and bad, and other polar opposites), it has no use for *neutrality*, (everything simply is). The mind is too limited a container for the vastness of Existence. A small cup cannot experience containing the whole ocean. The Divine may be an *idea in the mind*, but it will never be an *experience of the mind*. Therefore, we must rise above the mind to understand the true nature of our source and to view reality in its authentic totality. Only then can we identify with Pure Consciousness and fill the emptiness that aches in our soul.

Duality

The mind cannot possibly conceive or contain Universal Energy and accordingly does its best to interpret Existence through the tiny sphere of its own dualistic categorization system. After the mind has separated, labeled, grouped, and classified the information that it can grasp, it offers its own invention of reality in the form of divisions. We know such limitations as Good and Bad, Right and Wrong, God and Devil, Heaven and Hell, and other inventions of duality. The mind creates categories in order to build a recognizable structure, so that we can feel safe in the tiny tangible idea of life as we know it. The unlimited energy of Pure Consciousness, however, is not divisible. Similar to electricity, Pure Consciousness is neutral.

If we are unconscious in our actions, we may use electricity destructively and electrocute ourselves. If we advance with awareness and insight, we can apply electricity creatively to light a dark path. The energy itself is still neutral. We cannot divide it into good, bad, right, and wrong. How we utilize the energy determines the outcome.

Pure Consciousness is the electric energy flowing through us. Because we have free will, we can choose to use our power creatively or destructively. Consequently, our choices determine our life experience.

Our source is neutral.
The human mind is dualistic.

We live creativity when we align with the *neutral* essence of Pure Consciousness, while directing our thoughts and emotions (mind) consciously. We live destructively when we rely on the mind's *dualistic* system to determine our thoughts, emotions, and actions for us.

Similar to an automobile, the mind can help us move through time and space. When Pure Consciousness is in the driver's seat, it will direct the mind according to our dreams, wishes, inspirations, and intentions. When the mind is left to drive itself, however, it is likely to be distracted by any trivial outside influence and eventually end up in a ditch, leaving us with the uncomfortable feeling that we are not where we want to be in life.

The aspect of our being that has aspirations to evolve is not the mind. It is Pure Consciousness. The mind is simply a vehicle that contains tools, such as thoughts, ideas, and emotions, that act as fuel to keep it running. A positive life experience can only occur once we step into the driver's seat and direct the mind according to the inspiration of our soul.

Interpretations of Reality

Every mind that exists in the world has its own distorted interpretation of reality, based on its attachment to the duality with which it has aligned. Therefore, every mind looks out at a different world.

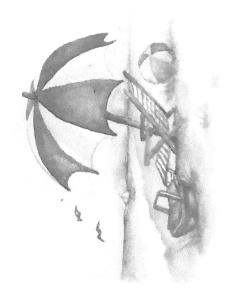

Dear Archie,

HAPPY NEW YEAR!!!!

Have not seen you in a while, but I think of you a lot and that always makes me smile. I hope all is well with you and your thriving practice and your happy volleyball days.

Forgive me for not writing to you more frequently. When I closed my practice a few years ago, I began devoting all of my time to working on a few projects, which took me away from the joy of writing to friends. But you are always in my heart and time away from those I love never puts a dint in anything for me.

Since you are such an avid reader and writer, I thought I would offer you this book. Wish I had come to you for editing, as I believe you would have done a much better job than the people I hired in L.A. Next time I will ask you first.

May 2008 be your most excellent and rewarding year yet.

Love and joy

Ehsida Bisset

Imagine two people out of the billions that exist. Each are wearing glasses tinted with a different impression of reality. One whose glasses are tinted with a calm reality, we will call Mr. Peace Seeker. One whose glasses are tinted with an angry reality, we will call Mr. Revenge. Mr. Peace Seeker sees the world with a peaceful hue covering it. Mr. Revenge sees the world with an angry haze covering it. Both of these fellows will be looking out at the same neutral world, but what they see will be entirely different.

Mr. Revenge will be convinced that the world is angry and filled with pain. He may even threaten to harm Mr. Peace Seeker if he refuses to agree with him. Mr. Peace Seeker might consider Mr. Revenge quite insane, since he could not imagine wanting to harm others. Mr. Peace Seeker and Mr. Revenge will frustrate each other whenever they come in contact, because their realities will feel so separate. The feeling of being separate leads to defensiveness, stress and falseness; all behaviors where destructive energy toward the self and others begins. If Mr. Peace Seeker and Mr. Revenge were to take their tainted glasses off, both of their realities would once again be seen as neutral, and they would be able to look out at the same world. Conflict only occurs when we are unable to drop our attachment to beliefs about right and wrong, good and bad, true and false, etc.

In this world, every mind is programmed with its own belief system, and everyone is certain that their perspective is the right one. This distortion of neutral energy is the cause of **all** dissension. In order to find a common ground for harmony and understanding, we must first take our dualistic glasses off by rising above the categorizations and limitations of the mind altogether.

Although it may appear that divergence is more prevalent between others, our greatest turbulence occurs because of the distorted view we have of ourselves. Once the mind has separated us from Pure Consciousness, it offers a perspective of the self that is worthless, unlovable, inadequate, insignificant, useless, unsafe, empty, deprived, out of control, powerless, not good enough, unstable, or bad.

As long as we identify with the mind, we will be led away from our original state of grace, and miss the experience of our neutral, unlimited, infinite, symbiotic, non-judgmental and boundless source.

What is the Mind?

Mind can be equated with a crowd of people at a party. Many ideas, opinions, and gossip fill the space—a chatterbox, commenting on everything it sees or hears; hundreds of voices all telling different stories; speaking over one another; drowning out the ability to make sense of anything.

Once a group of individuals disperse from a party, a crowd no longer exists. Once the thoughts within the mind disperse, mind no longer exists. What remains is Pure Consciousness.

The mind is not our most intelligent source, yet most people stop at the mind and search no further for greater knowing. They expect and are often taught that the mind is the ultimate vehicle for insight, solutions, and experience. This is not the case. When all thoughts disappear, there is a peaceful silence which opens the door to a much wiser and more evolved intelligence than the mind. We rarely connect with or listen to this inner wisdom, however, because we are in the habit of relying on the mind instead.

The mind is unable to grasp who we are in terms of energy, because it perceives life through corporeal reality; the tangible aspects of Existence. When we identify with the mind, anything intangible appears inconsequential or nonexistent. The blind man cannot conceive of light. The deaf man cannot conceive of sound, and the unconscious (mentally identified) man cannot conceive of Pure Consciousness flowing through his being.

Pure Consciousness is neither the mind nor the body. It is the energy flowing through everything, eager to guide us to our greatest heights.

What is Pure Consciousness?

Imagine for a moment that you have no responsibilities. You flow through life with no agenda, no judgments, no attachments, no rules, no bias, no obligations, no compromising, no duties or deadlines. There is no competition or comparison. *Everything simply…IS.*

Because you are completely free to flow and observe life from this neutral and unlimited place, exciting ideas begin to jump into your awareness. You see everything as energy, and you realize that your own *vibration* is the most powerful tool you have to make things happen. In fact, you are certain of your success, because you can feel the infinite power of your own Life Force.

Your experience is a free-flowing journey consisting of observing your environment from a neutral perspective, feeling the inspiration to add to what brings you joy, and playfully allowing your creations to form, with your happy, excited, high-vibrational energy.

In this pure reality, neutrality leads to freedom, expansion, and bliss. *Neutrality* is the beginning point or springboard into greater power and creativity. The neutral energy outlined above is a description of Pure Consciousness, which is pure, positive, creative energy with no attachments, no judgments, no agenda, and no ideas of good, bad, right, or wrong. With no attachments, nothing can hinder its flow, and the positive momentum of its force continues to grow.

This same creative energy flows through all of us and provides unlimited potential to expand with greater freedom, power, and bliss. We are 98% electric (Divine) energy. We are 2% physical. When we ignore the 98% by identifying only with the 2%, we deny most of our creative energy. Once we rise above the mind with all its attachments, identifications, categorizations, and judgments, we instantly become 98% more powerful.

When you accept the truth of your being, you will understand that a tremendous amount of action extended from your 2% physical self, has nowhere near the power of aligning with your pure, positive, creative 98% of self. Your electric vibration attracts and creates. Your 2% is insignificant in comparison.

In spite of this truth, the mind focuses 100% of our attention on the 2% of our reality, which is only the beginning of how the mind limits our power and understanding of self.

How the Mind is Formed

The mind is like litmus paper; every impression has left a mark. The ideas, praise, and punishments of parents, the preaching of religious leaders, basic societal beliefs, schooling, literature, television, media, entertainment, computers, peer group banter, relatives, siblings, friends, political dominance during childhood, and how the individual responded to or interpreted information—comprises the mind. It is a compilation of ideas, rules, categories, limitations, and opinions formed by the masses who have failed to align with Pure Consciousness before we arrived.

In our youth, we are initially more in touch with the positive, playful energy of our source, but as we rely on our surroundings for physical survival, the voice of parents, teachers, acquaintances, and friends all begin to carry more authority than our own inner knowing. These outside conjectures are recorded by our psyche and play over and over again like a broken record in our mind.

Children's original connection to Pure Consciousness becomes clouded as they learn to perceive life through the mind and they begin to follow along with the crowd. Eventually, a child will forget their *true self* and instead react to the world from the perspective of their programmed mind or ego personality, which is all a projected illusion created by society.

The Mind Has the Power to Project Any Illusion

The mind itself is a dream. As long as we identify with the mind, we are cooperating with any illusion it projects.

In the morning we may wake up from our dreams, but we are still in the mind, so another sort of dream continues. In fact, the mind has even more control over us during the day than it does at night while we sleep and dream.

When the anorexic look at their reflection in a mirror, their minds project an obese image over their true physique, so they will continue on with the pattern of starving themselves to death. Similarly, the depressed mind will project a gloomy veil over everything in life so that nothing is able to stimulate joy or satisfaction. Also, the prejudice mind can assume an injustice that instigates rage even under the most innocent or non-biased conditions.

Along with visual and cognitive deceptions, any negative banter the mind offers about how inadequate we are, will appear valid to us when we identify with its programming. These distortions are based on the mind's inability to see the greater truth of our being.

We rely on the mind the most when we are under stress; exactly the time when we must reach for a higher source of intelligence. The mind has no ability to offer us legitimate solutions to our agony or trauma; it will superimpose an illusion to keep us unconscious instead.

Thirsty travelers in a burning desert will be offered a mirage of waterfalls that do not exist as a solution to dehydration, urging sojourners deeper into the fiery plane to appease their thirst. Similarly, a hurt or stressed ego will seek an avenue of escape—for example, blaming someone else—which will cause the individual to venture deeper into denial, resentment, and conflict. In this manner, the mind will project solutions to our fears and traumas that lead us in the direction of more pain and emptiness, instead of offering true resolution.

For twenty-four hours every day the mind fills our imagination with fears, negative beliefs, and limited ideas, all of which we assume are real. We cooperate with these illusions unconsciously, because we have no reason to question the validity of the mind's projections, just as we feel no need to question the images in our dreams. Only when we wake up to a more poignant reality do we realize everything we believed was merely an illusion.

Until you raise your level of consciousness, you will not know what is a projection of the mind and what is reality. The mind itself is a dream, and we must awaken the dreamer.

The Basic Structure of the Mind

The structure of the mind is formed around dividing and categorizing all experiences in order to build a base of certainty about life. If the mind can condemn something as bad or recognize something as good, it feels secure and empowered. Compartmentalizing is its comfort and identity. Conversely, if the mind cannot find a category for something, it remains disturbed and immobilized.

The following ideas make up the basic structure of the mind:

• Time and Space
• Life and Death
• Matter and Energy
• Physical Proof and Imagination
• Positive and Negative

In order to compartmentalize reality, the mind forms these concepts into various dualities, such as:

- Right and Wrong
- Good and Bad
- Moral and Immoral
- Innocence and Guilt
- God and Devil
- True and False
- Powerful and Weak
- Rich and Poor
- Useful and Burden
- Safe and Unsafe
- Stable and Unstable
- Peace and Disharmony
- Order and Chaos

These dualities form such emotions as:

- Infatuation and Hate
- Serenity and Anger
- Joy and Sorrow

When you find yourself identifying with these dualities, you are aligning with the mind's distorted view of a neutral reality. Separation only exists within the structure of our belief systems. All things more powerful than we are exist without any need for categorizing. The earth, the sun, the moon, and all of nature live free from the duality of the mind. The Universe thrives on neutrality, which leads to greater creativity, expansion, and joy. The mind thrives on duality, which leads to judgment, pain, and destruction.

What is the Ego?

When the mind becomes identified with its determinations of good, bad, right, and wrong, it first forms fears about these identifications, and then it complicates itself by adding an ego. The ego fights to protect and defend itself from its imagined fears. Ego formation is the root or catalyst of all emotional pain.

If the mind is likened to a crowd, than the ego can be compared to someone to whom we are attached in that crowd. If you see strangers in a group holding hands with each other, you may have no reaction at all. If you see your lover in a crowd holding hands with someone new, however, you *will* experience a reaction. The ego forms attachments and strong identifications with ideas about reality. Then it reacts defensively to these ideas. The painful response you may have watching your lover hold hands with a new person, is entirely due to the attachments of the ego.

How is the Ego Formed?

Core fears that the mind assumes during childhood form the basis of the ego structure and cause a fear-based outlook on life. Our potential to create and live joyfully is diminished, because the ego focuses most of our attention and energy on defending against imagined fears.

Nine core fears form nine basic ego structures within humanity:

1)   The fear of being bad

2)   The fear of being unwanted or unworthy of love

3)   The fear of not being enough

4)   The fear of having no purpose or significance

5) The fear of applying personal power (incapable)

6) The fear of being unsafe or unstable without outside support

7) The fear of loss and deprivation

8) The fear of being vulnerable or unprotected (no control)

9) The fear of being disturbed or in pain

The Nine Basic Ego Structures

1) The person whose ego is formed around the *fear of being bad* will believe they must redeem themselves from their imagined *sins* in order to appear good. They often live by a set of rigid rules they hope will prove their own righteousness. Frequently, they seek out others who do not align with these rules in order to expose them for their sins and point the finger away from themselves, thereby avoiding the condemnation they believe they deserve deep down.

2) The person whose ego is formed around the *fear of being unworthy of love* will desperately seek love and approval from the outer world, often becoming a predator for sex, attention, or pity. To appear worthy of love, they may live a life of service and sacrifice themselves for any cause that might illuminate their selfless actions, as they hope to appear to be the *most* worthy of love in the eyes of society.

3) The person whose ego is formed around the *fear of not being enough* will become aggressively competitive and try to prove they are better than everyone else. They strive to win at any cost, even to the point of the obliteration of those who appear better than they are. If they are unable to impress others or reach the success they desire, they will cheat, lie, steal, or assume someone else's important image. In extreme cases, the mind will superimpose a narcissistic view of the self and treat others as peons.

4) The person whose ego is formed around the *fear of having no purpose or significance* will need an extraordinary amount of attention and emotional support in order to feel worthy of being alive. Their ego constantly reminds them that their accomplishments are insignificant compared to what they are required to achieve. If they do not receive the unconditional support or praise they desire, they fall into depression and blame the world for their pain and suffering, often remaining stuck in the woes of their past. Pointing out everything negative about life and everything they hate about others can become their chosen *purpose* in order to feel powerful or significant.

5) The person whose ego is formed around the *fear of applying their own power* will find it difficult or unpleasant interacting with intimidating or aggressive people, because they fear they may be overpowered or manipulated in some way. Without the application of their own power, they begin to see themselves as useless or incapable in a world driven by aggression and force. Eventually they may close down to society altogether, often becoming reclusive in order to avoid the possibility of anyone taking liberties with their sacred space or personal boundaries.

6) The person whose ego is formed around the *fear of not being able to remain safe or secure on their own* will often dread responsibility and become homeless or put up with abusive relationships in order to have a place to live or work. Their ego constantly reminds them they cannot accomplish anything all on their own, which makes them feel the need to depend on groups, family structures, religious or political organizations, friends, committed partners, clubs or communities for their feelings of safety and structure. This dependence eventually leads to greater insecurity as well as resentment.

7) The person whose ego is formed around the *fear of loss and deprivation* will be insatiable for immediate gratification and become

reckless with their finances, relationships, and health. Their ego continually generates fear that they will be deprived of the high levels of excitement and attention they desire, or that they will eventually lose the source of joy and stimulation on which they rely.

8) The person whose ego is formed around the *fear of being unprotected* will aggressively dominate, intimidate, control, and harm others as a means to protect themselves. When they have a desire to love someone, the ego will convince them that no one is safe to love, so their heart remains closed as a protective measure.

9) The person whose ego is formed around the *fear of pain or disharmony* may live in their own private fantasy world where they can pretend pain and disharmony do not exist. Every time they begin to acknowledge their need for action, the ego will distract them with a fantasy so they can prolong avoiding their painful circumstances. This personality has severe resistance to change.

All ego personalities cause distorted motivations and cruel or pathetic behavior. The basis of the ego structure will shape a personality into something far from what nature intended and block the true magnificence of our soul.

The Nine Basic Soul Essences

Introducing the Magnificence of each Soul

Our planet is comprised of elements which in unity make up a whole. Pure Consciousness is also made up of qualities which form together to create what we call *Existence* or *Universal Energy*. Nine basic ingredients maintain a cosmic balance:

1) ORDER

2) LOVE

3) GROWTH

4) SPIRIT

5) TRUTH

6) STABILITY

7) ECSTASY

8) POWER

9) PEACE

Every *being* on earth enters as a representative of one of these essences. This, our Soul Essence, makes up the Spiritual DNA of our soul and determines our specific drive or motivation in life.

These basic essences or spirit groups translate into life purposes or intentions of the soul.

1)   ORDER *(Harmony, Organization, Regulation)*

Those entering with the essence of ORDER will feel an intrinsic drive to create order within society. Often such individuals gravitate toward the fields of law, religion, politics, corrections, enforcement, education, architecture, banking, directing or sanitation. They choose areas that will help them discourage unruliness and encourage justice. At their peak, they are capable of setting standards and guidelines which enhance society and increase the goodness in mankind. The Declaration of Independence, written by Thomas Jefferson; whose essence was ORDER, exemplifies this universal energy. Clint Eastwood, Frank Lloyd Wright, George Washington, Krishnamurti, Nelson Mandela, and Patanjali are other inspirational individuals who have reached great heights expressing the essence of ORDER.

2) LOVE *(Oneness, Unity, Marriage)*

Those entering with the essence of LOVE will feel driven toward nurturing others as well as creating bonds and unity within society. Often this inspires individuals toward the healing arts, child care, teaching, aesthetic fields, counseling, family planning, communications, or animal care. At their peak, they exude unconditional love, which nourishes and inspires everyone on their path. Jesus is a good example of an individual who exemplified the essence of LOVE. In doing so, he inspired many to love more deeply and generously as well. Doreen Virtue, Esther Hicks, Louise L. Hay, Meera, Mother Teresa, and Princess Diana are other inspirational people who have reached great heights expressing the essence of LOVE.

3) GROWTH *(Material Manifestation, Expansiveness, Transformation)*

Those entering with the essence of GROWTH will be highly motivated and energetic. They are eager to make a difference, manifest abundance and reach some peak of excellence within their chosen field. Those infused with the essence of GROWTH are often drawn toward big business ventures, self-help organizations, athletics, high-profile venues including acting, modeling or politics, as well as social fields where interaction with others is predominant. At their peak, they are able to motivate and inspire others to transform, improve, grow, reach greater heights, and continue to excel in life. Moses is a good example of an individual who exemplified the essence of GROWTH. Arnold Schwarzenegger, Jack Canfield, Oprah Winfrey, Shirley MacLaine, Tom Cruise, and Tony Robbins are other inspirational people who have reached great heights expressing the essence of GROWTH.

4) SPIRIT *(Emotional Expression, Life, Divinity)*

Those entering with the essence of SPIRIT are driven by their emotions and their need to express their feelings in a creative form. Their motivation generates a very sensitive nature, which promotes excellence in the fields of acting, poetry, singing, dancing, writing, romancing, drawing, painting, designing, and interacting with others in an in-depth and emotional way. At their peak, they are able to inspire a connection to spirit in those who open to their gifts. Krishna is a good example of an individual who exemplified the essence of SPIRIT. Hermann Hesse, Edgar Degas, Johnny Depp, Michael Jackson, The artist formerly known as Prince, and Sinead O'Connor are other inspirational people who have reached great heights expressing the essence of SPIRIT.

5)   TRUTH *(Understanding, Depth of Experience, Awareness)*

Those entering with the essence of TRUTH seek a depth of experience which leads to profound knowledge and visionary perception. Their keen minds may become intrigued with research, science, metaphysics, physics, psychiatry, writing, and mathematics. Some may even share their profound insights through an art form. At their peak, they are able to convey complicated matter in simplistic style for the benefit of all. Socrates and Lao Tzu are good examples of individuals who exemplified the essence of TRUTH. Albert Einstein, George Lucas, J. K. Rowling, John Lennon, Leonardo Da Vinci, and Stephen Hawking are other inspirational people who have reached great heights expressing the essence of TRUTH.

6)   STABILITY *(Structure, Reliability, Responsibility)*

Those entering with the essence of STABILITY are driven toward building a community, family, organization, system, or support group which uplifts and enhances society. Drawn to the fields of higher education, politics, theater, music, numbers and religion, they seek to create a stable ground which will offer greater support for others to flourish. At their peak, they establish structures which encourage interest in the joy of living instead of the struggle for survival. Pythagoras and Rajneesh are good examples of individuals who exemplified the essence of STABILITY. Billy Crystal, Robert Kennedy, Ron Howard, Susan Sarandan, Tom Hanks and Will Smith are other inspirational people who have reached great heights expressing the essence of STABILITY.

7)   ECSTASY *(Creativity, Fulfillment, Emotions of Elation)*

Those entering with the essence of ECSTASY are driven toward excitement, often finding themselves in the limelight due to their outrageous creativity and outspokenness. These individuals yearn to entertain, tickle, and uplift others with their genius minds and seemingly inexhaustible energy. At their peak, they lighten up the planet with their brilliance and inventiveness, inspiring others to laugh and celebrate life at each moment. Mozart is a good example of an individual who reached a Divine link with the essence of ECSTASY, allowing it to filter through his music and uplift the masses. Goldie Hawn, Michelangelo Buonarroti, J.R.R. Tolkien, Robin Williams, Shakespeare and Steven Spielberg are other inspirational people who have reached great heights expressing the essence of ECSTASY.

8)   POWER *(Energy, Effectiveness and Abundance)*

Those entering with the essence of POWER are highly motivated to inspire others to use and apply their own power. Often drawn toward heading large enterprises that employ or support others, this group yearns to safeguard and empower everyone. At their peak, they create a protective shield around those for whom they care, as well as the planet at large. They spread their unparalleled love and compassion out to the masses with extraordinary generosity and leadership. George Gurdjieff is a good example of an individual who exemplified the essence of POWER. Angelina Jolie, Indira Gandhi, Lee Iacocca, Martin Luther King Jr., Theodore Roosevelt and Winston Churchill are other inspirational people who have reached great heights expressing the essence of POWER.

9) PEACE *(Stillness, Tranquility, Serenity)*

Those entering with the essence of PEACE yearn to create harmony and serenity everywhere they go. Drawn to the healing arts, entertainment, religious fields, music, writing, environmental causes, and other graceful endeavors, they soothe the atmosphere with their profound sense of inner peace and wisdom. Buddha is a good example of an individual who exemplified the essence of PEACE. Abraham Lincoln, Deepak Chopra, Jimmy Stewart, Mikhail Gorbachev, Peace Pilgrim, and Walt Disney are other inspirational people who have reached great heights expressing the essence of PEACE.

As children we exude our true essence freely, but as the ego forms and the personality takes over, we begin to feel separate from our essence and consequently live contrary to our purpose.

SOUL ESSENCE	EGO PERSONALITY
1) ORDER	*1) CHAOS*
2) LOVE	*2) SEPARATENESS*
3) GROWTH	*3) DESTRUCTION*
4) SPIRIT	*4) VOID*
5) TRUTH	*5) ILLUSION*
6) STABILITY	*6) INSTABILITY*
7) ECSTASY	*7) EMPTINESS*
8) POWER	*8) INEFFECTIVENESS*
9) PEACE	*9) DISTURBANCE*

1) The essence of ORDER, which aspires to create only good, will be blocked by the ego's core *fear of being bad,* and create *CHAOS* as a result.

2) The essence of LOVE, which aspires toward unity, will be blocked by the ego's core *fear of being unworthy of love*, causing the experience of *SEPARATION*.

3) The essence of GROWTH, which aspires toward creative expansion, will be blocked by the ego's core *fear of failure, or of not being good enough*, causing decline and a personality which is *DESTRUCTIVE*.

4) The essence of SPIRIT, which aspires toward inspirational expression, becomes blocked by the ego's core *fear of having no purpose*, causing a feeling of *VOID* or insignificance.

5) The essence of TRUTH, which aspires toward Divine understanding, becomes blocked by the ego's core *fear of being unable to apply one's power*, causing disparaging thinking, which leads to *ILLUSIONS*.

6) The essence of STABILITY, which aspires toward building solid structures, will be blocked by the ego's core *fear of being unsafe and unstable*, causing *INSTABILITY*.

7) The essence of ECSTASY, which aspires toward fulfillment, will be blocked by the ego's core *fear of loss and deprivation*, causing a feeling of *EMPTINESS*.

8) The essence of POWER, which aspires toward protecting and empowering others, becomes blocked by the ego's core *fear of being vulnerable to harm*, causing *INEFFECTIVENESS*.

9) The essence of PEACE, which aspires toward creating harmony, becomes blocked by the ego's core *fear of being in pain*, causing *DISTURBANCE*.

To live authentically, we must rise above the ego's core fear and align once again with our original essence. Only then are we capable of receiving the fulfillment we yearn for in life. The first criteria toward evolution is to know and see clearly who and what we are, first as a personality and then more deeply as a representative of Existence here to express the truth of our soul.

When is the Ego in Control?

Ego is the only cause of pain and suffering. If we are not in a state of pure love and ecstasy, we are processing life through the ego. We may blame our pain on others, but blame itself is a function of the ego. The ego creates many characteristics that you might recognize immediately. It causes us to hate, argue, gossip, condemn, judge, belittle, abuse, betray, worry, obsess, and compete, etc. The ego instigates defensiveness, addictions, weakness, shame, sadness, victimhood, martyrdom, dependencies, deprivation, lust, jealousy, infatuation, neediness, phobias, neurosis, narcissism, limitations, purpose-lessness, panic, instability, insincerity, scatteredness, insanity, manic behavior, depression, controlling or manipulative tendencies, and escapism.

According to the ego, happiness lies outside of the self, because *the self is the problem*. People who continually reach out to others for love, approval, compliments, attention, affection, support, safety, escape, security, and a feeling of belonging, control or self-importance, are the people most burdened by the hungry ego.

A particularly dangerous aspect of the ego is deception. It hides the existence of Pure Consciousness from us in every possible way. Most people have no idea that anything like Pure Consciousness exists, that it is easily accessible to all of us, or that it is the most significant ingredient that makes up who we are.

Why Does the Ego Exist?

Some may ask, "What purpose does the ego serve?"

Other than giving us a structure in which to believe and a false identity, the ego exists to create a distinction. Ego demonstrates the experience of being disconnected from Pure Consciousness. Once a fish has been out of water, it has a greater respect and appreciation for its true home in the sea. Land creates a clear distinction for the fish, just as ego creates a clear distinction for our soul.

When we perceive life through our core fear or ego, we experience dissatisfaction everywhere we turn. Eternal fulfillment can only be found by re-connecting with our source. We must rise above the ego in order to merge with the infinite power of Pure Consciousness. The discontent that ego generates inspires us toward this transformation.

Transformation

"Nothing is ever destroyed, it only changes form."
—EINSTEIN

Everything is always in a state of growth and expansion. A flower was once a seed, then a sprout, then a beautiful celebration of blooming color. Beyond this stage, she becomes fragrant and spreads out farther than her petals can extend with an exotic scent.

When the flower has reached the highest level of evolution as a flower, her flesh moves back into the earth, and her fragrance travels on—continuing to expand, advance and grow. Nothing ever comes to an end energetically—it simply goes on changing form.

Having an ego is the seed stage in humanity. We must pass beyond this stagnant phase for our essence to bloom. Our essence is Pure Consciousness, which is a highly evolved aspect of the ego, just as the fragrance of a flower is the highly evolved aspect of the seed.

Those who hold on tightly to the ego limit their power and remain at a lower vibration. They never allow themselves to enjoy the amazing beauty of life. Without this transformation, their energy turns destructive. Those who transform their ego, increase in power and naturally become more creative.

We do not want to battle the ego. We want to understand its qualities and use them to our advantage. With a greater understanding of the ego, and a greater awareness of our Soul Essence, we are more equipped to rise above the limitations of the ego and open to our true power.

In order to rise above the ego, we must first become aware of it. This process of viewing the ego is made possible through *The Witnessing Technique.*

CHAPTER 2

The Witnessing Technique

Introduction

THE FIRST STEP BEYOND THE MIND is to begin observing your thoughts. Once you become the witness of your thoughts, the programming in the mind can no longer determine your behavior. The Witnessing Technique bypasses the need to psychoanalyze the mind, because the mind is not you. All you must do is learn to stand apart from the mind. With this approach you can observe the mind's actions, watch its behavior and realize that the aspect of your consciousness that is able to witness and be aware of the mind, is the wiser, stronger part of your being.

The Witnessing Self

The mind cannot observe itself. Only the *witnessing aspect* of our consciousness can watch the mind. This *Witnessing Self* is our direct connection to Pure Consciousness.

A Picture Speaks a Thousand Words

Having the patience to observe the thoughts in the mind can be a frustrating task at first. Before long most people grow bored, become discouraged, or fall asleep. Not only is this a difficult exercise, but the deeper beliefs and patterns which lead to destructive behavior are often disguised by familiarity. The Witnessing Technique will access these more complicated patterns through the use of symbolism.

Our mind communicates innate meaning through pictures. The faces of loved ones have a greater impact on us than a sentence that describes them. The symbols or images we find in the mind represent our programmed thoughts, feelings, and beliefs. Our subconscious and conscious beliefs about ourselves determine our behavior.

If you are reading a children's book written in ancient Sanskrit, you may not understand the words, but the pictures could help you determine the basic story line. Often the sporadic thoughts we find in our mind won't make much sense to us either, but when we allow our emotions to form into images which represent our thoughts and feelings, a story about our programming will begin to unfold. The *Witnessing Technique* is based on the use of these inner pictures or symbols in order to access the deeper programming within the mind.

Once you learn how to access the images within your mind, viewing your subconscious becomes as simple as watching a movie, and it is often quite entertaining. After a while you will notice archetypes which clearly represent how your mind is programmed to react to life. One helpful path to the symbolism is to begin with a strong emotion which has surfaced while under stress.

Stress Reveals our Programming

Under stress we respond to life via our core fear and programmed ideas of good, bad, right, wrong. If we see someone doing something the mind has determined is wrong and bad, or right and good, the ego forms a strong emotional response to it. Everyone experiences their own unique reaction to stress, based on the core fear around which their personality has formed and their specific ideas of good, bad, right, and wrong.

An individual who is aggressively cut off in traffic may become empowered by the challenge of a competition on the road. If their core fear is based in not feeling important enough, they will be driven to compete to prove their superiority to the other drivers. The right thing to do, according to this individual's programming, may be to chase the aggressive motorist down and cut him or her off in order to get even.

Another individual in the same situation may become nervous or frightened. If they have a core fear of applying their own power, they will view all the assertive drivers as more powerful than they are and find themselves becoming timid, worried, and overly cautious. This person's programming may tell him or her that the right thing to do is move over to the slow lane and go thirty miles per hour to avoid any further danger.

Someone driving behind the timid motorist may become frustrated and jump to the conclusion that others are always getting in their way and slowing them down. If their core fear is based in feeling vulnerable to harm, they will be driven to gain control over the situation in order to protect themselves. The right thing to do, according to their programming, may be to honk their horn and tailgate the slower motorist until they intimidate them off the road. In this manner, their ego feels they have exerted control over the situation.

Others may go home and kick the dog, beat their spouse, scream at the children, watch television, eat junk food, get drunk, take drugs, or go on a shopping spree to feel better. These responses are sparked by their core fear. Our core fears and the ideas we hold about what is good, bad, right, and wrong, make up our own unique mental programming, which forms the foundation of our personalities and, therefore, our actions.

Most of our programming instigates momentary insanity during times of intense stress, causing people to feel validated in abusing, killing, punishing, betraying, condemning, controlling, confronting, blaming, and harming themselves and others. To move beyond our negative programming, we must learn to stand apart from the mind and identify instead with our *Witnessing Self*.

Dealing with Stress

People have been taught two ways of dealing with painful emotions. The first and most common way is to *express* it and take it out on someone else. The second way is to *suppress* the energy and allow it to implode on the self. Neither of these choices will transform the pain, which is bound to occur again and again and build momentum as time goes on.

There is a third way of dealing with painful emotions which does not involve suppression or explosion. When a negative emotion arises we can transform the energy through The Witnessing Technique. We *witness* the energy by allowing the **emotion itself** to form into an image which represents it. Then we allow the image in our imagination to act out the emotion for us, while we observe from the neutral perspective of our *Witnessing Self*.

The emotion is processed in a safe and thorough way, as the character or image is given free rein to act out the emotional energy until it has dissolved. By allowing the image unlimited freedom to go wild, (with the emotion it represents), it will eventually act out our pain and aggression within the safety of our own imagination.

As we watch the characters behavior, we are observing a symbolic representation of our programmed beliefs. When we identify with the *witnessing* aspect of our consciousness, we are building the awareness that we are **not** the programming. *We are the observer of it.*

Once we reach a sense of calm or neutrality about the emotion, we can easily rise above the programming in the mind which ignites our suffering. As an alternative, we can identify more significantly with the witnessing aspect of our consciousness, and simply observe with no attachment to the pain. The same tumultuous emotion is less likely to occur as we become more conscious of the programming which causes it.

As our identification with Pure Consciousness strengthens, we will be aware of emotional energy, but it will no longer have control over our lives. As the witness, we can choose our own responses and direct our thoughts instead of relying on the mind to determine our behavior and point of focus for us.

Beginning the Technique

A good place to begin the technique is to identify a specific emotion that surfaced during a recent stressful event.

Emotional Symbolism

Close your eyes and find the strongest emotion which captures your reaction to the stressful event. As an example, let's imagine that you discover anger. Allow your anger to be present and sense what the anger feels like. Is it sharp, stabbing, hot, burning, dull, or explosive? Does it appear as a specific color, shape, character, size, or texture? Allow the qualities of what you are experiencing to emerge as an image which best represents the intensity of the emotion. Do not force this to happen. Instead, simply allow your feelings to guide the image into form.

The emotion may turn into a human character, an animal, a cartoon character, an archetypal image, or a vision of energy. Even some sort of nothingness, such as a blank screen or an empty room may appear. Trust whatever comes forward, and then make sure it actually represents the emotion that you are feeling.

Once the emotion itself has taken a visual form in your mind, observe what the image does to express the feeling it represents. Watch carefully and do not attempt to direct or change it in any way. Allow it free rein over how it wants to express the emotion.

Just as you might watch two actors arguing in a film, watch the chaos in the mind with detached alertness and understand that the real you, *The Witness*, has nothing to do with the ego's pandemonium.

For an example, we take a look at a man from California named Ryan.

Ryan had a growing rage over the motorists he encountered on his morning journey into downtown Los Angeles. Whenever he thought about the people who cut in front of him, his heart would begin to race, his face would turn red, his breathing would grow heavy, and he would burst into a violent commentary, threatening to kill the next motorist who sped in front of him.

When he was guided to close his eyes and allow the intensity of his rage to form into an image, the vision of an angry King Kong appeared. King Kong expressed the rage in his imagination by moving through the busy freeway pounding on all the cars that had cut him off. Sometimes the image of King Kong would select a specific car, pick it up and growl at the driver, then rip the car apart or hurl it hard against a building.

Ryan watched the image of King Kong vent his rage until he felt quite calm. His rage was transformed by the character within the safety of his own imagination and within a few minutes, he was able to reflect on the drivers who had cut him off and remain neutral.

Once he felt neutral, he was guided to identify with the aspect of his consciousness that had been able to observe King Kong in his mind. As soon as he identified with his *Witnessing Self*, he felt peaceful, empowered, and capable of focusing his awareness on uplifting, creative things, instead of brooding on his pain.

As Ryan continued to identify with higher levels of consciousness, he discovered that he could step aside from his rage and observe the fury of King Kong as if the anger had nothing to do with him. *By watching King Kong, Ryan was watching his subconscious beliefs about himself and the programming which had instructed him to respond with anger.*

Once Ryan reached this level of awareness, he was able to observe clearly what his mind had been programmed to do under stress. As he continued to watch the image, he realized that the King Kong character attacked the cars, because he was afraid the drivers had been attacking him. King Kong interpreted these attacks to mean that the other drivers thought he was bad and wrong. He took it personally when people cut in front of him, assuming they were trying to punish him.

By watching his image more closely, Ryan realized that he had a core fear that he was bad. Anytime he felt punished, he would fly into a rage and accuse his perpetrator of being wrong and bad in order to defend himself against his own fear of being bad. This same programming showed up in many aspects of Ryan's life.

Prior to practicing The Witnessing Technique, Ryan's desire to vent his pain and appease his fear of being bad, caused him to follow motorists until they parked and got out of their cars. Then he would jump out of his truck and scream at them until he felt they had received an adequate reprimand. According to his programming, he had to make the other drivers admit they were the bad ones, so that he could feel redeemed in his own mind.

Ryan's mental programming was not giving him a real solution to his pain. His rage not only recurred, but also grew with intensity. As he continued to encounter more aggressive drivers, he experienced more hopelessness, frustration and anger. After a while, he felt he was ready to kill the people who cut in front of him. He was becoming the very thing that he strove to fight against.

This is exactly what the ego does to us. *We become what we fear when our programming is in control.*

Most of society responds to stress in a similar manner. The average mind will urge an individual to fight against their fears and those who cause them to surface. Inevitably, such an approach only increases the amount of control their fears have over them. Hence, they attract more circumstances which ignite more fear.

When we become the *witness*, however, we lift our focus away from the fear and direct it toward the innately peaceful aspect of our being, which remains neutral as it **calmly observes** the fearful programming. *How we view ourselves has everything to do with how we perceive others, as well as their reactions to us.*

As Ryan continued to practice The Witnessing Technique, he became capable of remaining neutral each time he felt anger arise. *He neither suppressed the anger nor expressed it. He observed it.* As he watched King Kong act out the intensity of his emotions for him, his anger transformed.

The Witnessing Technique has an alchemical effect on all negative emotions. Within a very short time, compulsive emotions that have dominated your interactions will no longer be able to deplete you or influence regrettable behavior. When Ryan chose to witness his pattern with rage, instead of allowing his programming to manipulate him, his commute to work became a pleasant drive, instead of a battlefield where his ego exercised control over him.

Overview

Once you find the symbol which represents your emotion, simply watch the image while it expresses your emotion until you feel indifferent or at peace. Then become aware of the *viewing aspect* of your consciousness that is able to observe the image. This *neutral* part of you that is able to *witness* the image **without emotional attachment** is Pure Consciousness. Know yourself as that.

As stress occurs, continue to allow your emotions to be expressed through the images they form in your mind. Anchor the awareness that you are not the image or the emotion. *YOU* are the neutral *witness* of these things.

Witnessing Steps

1. Find a strong emotion you want to transform.

2. Allow the emotion to take the form of an image which best represents it.

3. Permit the image to express itself with intense totality in your imagination.

4. Observe what happens without choreographing the actions.

5. Continue to watch the image until the emotion has lost its charge.

6.   Once you reach a feeling of neutrality about the emotion, you will be able to leave the pain with the image. When this shift occurs, become aware of the aspect of your consciousness that is able to *observe* the image.

7.   *Identify* with the observant aspect of your consciousness.

8.   Luxuriate in the empowering feeling of aligning with your *Witnessing Self,* instead of remaining trapped in the pain of the image.

After you have experienced the higher perspective of your Witnessing Self, determine what aspect of your mental programming your image symbolizes. By doing this, you will recognize how you respond to specific thoughts and emotions under stress. Once you become aware of how your mind chooses to react, you will be more capable of witnessing your emotions, instead of turning into them.

The Image Represents the Programming

As long as you are in the neutral position of watching the mind, your programming cannot force you to act out a destructive emotion. When Ryan became aware of King Kong, he was not about to become him. The insane emotions of the characters appear absurd to the Witnessing Self, but they seem perfectly rational to the mind. Remember—they were the mind's idea in the first place. Ryan was supposed to turn into an angry King Kong, because his mind determined that this would be the right thing to do when people made him feel bad.

Do not be afraid to admit the worst or ugliest programming you find within yourself. Everyone will feel a little silly once they see what their mind has been forcing them to do. Identifying the programming is important, so that you can avoid letting the mind take over in the future. The more you witness your programming, the funnier it becomes and the less likely you are to take the projected pain of the ego seriously.

The character or image into which the emotion forms will show you a symbolic representation of how your programming controls you. The person holding a rageful King Kong type programming, will be much like King Kong when they are angry. The programming in their mind will urge them to act out with barbaric behavior, which will motivate merciless punishment of others. The more you can discover about your images, the more power you will have over your programming.

As Ryan continued to watch his destructive image, he recognized that King Kong believed he was an authority figure over others. Ryan had a core fear that he was bad, so his personality was formed around trying to prove that he was not only good, but also more noble than anyone else. This idea was the foundation of his personality, so he was not consciously aware of how his actions appeared until he began to watch the image of King Kong.

In order to hide his fear of being bad, Ryan's mind superimposed the idea that he was righteous and that everyone else was bad, which was what he believed when things were going well. Under stress, however, his core fear of being bad would surface, creating a need to prove to others that he was good, while forcing them to admit they were bad.

According to Ryan's programming, society was supposed to bow down to his demands immediately and receive his reprimands, which were based on his own internal rule or law. When he took a deeper look at this illusion, he understood how outrageous it was, even if his ego still wished it were true.

Transformation

Ryan began to witness the King Kong character every time he felt himself become angry or punitive. He understood that the cause of his anger arose from the need to defend his saint-like image and prove he was innocent and good. That was the root of all his anger.

Please understand the importance of this. If you watch your programming, you will discover that you have **one specific core fear** that will be the catalyst for all your emotions. Your personality (how you respond to the world) is formed as a reaction to your core fear.

Ryan's fear of being bad was also the stimulating factor every time he felt depressed, hopeless, and ashamed. His positive emotions were inspired by the feeling that others perceived him as good. Once you are able to recognize your own core fear, you will have a better understanding of why your mind causes you to react the way you do to life. More importantly, you will have the power to witness your fears, instead of falling victim to them.

Once Ryan had risen above his core fear, he no longer felt defensive or insulted when other motorists cut in front of him. Instead, he felt compassion for the aggressive drivers, knowing they must be trapped in their own torture chamber of mental programming.

The ego is a projection of false ideas. The Witnessing Self reflects only what is real. Transformation is as simple as seeing the truth. Your true self is overflowing with love, goodness, power, creativity, and joy. As you identify with your Witnessing Self, these attributes are what you will find.

Your alignment with Pure Consciousness must become your state of being in order for you to respond to the world as this euphoric energy. Otherwise, your will remain trapped in the inept, unloved, worthless idea of self the mind has projected for you.

Common Challenges

Beginning the Technique

For those who are heavily identified with the ego, The Witnessing Technique will appear too simple and the mind will want to think its way through each step instead of allowing an experience to take place. The ego will also want to complicate things by trying to change the image or choreograph the behavior.

The following example demonstrates common challenges a controlling mind will have with The Witnessing Technique. Much like Ryan with his King Kong character, the following individual suffers from the core fear of being bad. You will notice that even though both people share the same core fear, their behavior is still uniquely their own, based on their specific ideas about good, bad, right, and wrong.

Tony is a good example of an individual who is heavily identified with a defensive ego.

Tony was a police officer who was experiencing a lot of difficulty with his superiors at work. When he began The Witnessing Technique, he found an image that represented his core fear of being bad. The vision that appeared for Tony was a dog in his dog house digging in the dirt. He was a bad dog, and he was sent to his dog house because he had done something wrong. The dog expressed his feelings of frustration by throwing dirt in the air. As Tony described the image, it became apparent to him that the dog felt he was doing everything wrong, and that he would get in trouble no matter how hard he tried to do everything right.

Tony was guided to observe the image of the dog, who he named Rex, until he felt neutral about the emotion Rex represented. Tony was adamant, however, that he had to change Rex into a good dog first. Because of his desire to fix the dog, Tony was unwilling to reach a neutral detached experience. As a result, he was unable to identify with his Witnessing Self.

Crucial to the technique, one must understand that the image appearing in the mind is only a representation of the programming. It is not supposed to change or improve or come to any conclusions. Rex the bad dog simply represents the programming of feeling wrong and bad in Tony's mind. In order for Tony to rise above his painful programming, he would have to rise above the image of Rex the dog and observe him from a neutral perspective. As long as he remains identified with Rex the dog and tries to fix and improve him, he will remain attached to the idea of being wrong and bad.

Remember that Witnessing is not about changing the programming in the mind. The intent of Witnessing is to **view the programming, then rise above it.**

Leave the Emotion with the Image

The emotion and the image are attached to each other. The image represents the pain of the emotion. You are not the emotion. The character in your image is. Leave the emotion behind with the character and observe from a distance. Allow the image to feel the intensity of the emotion by itself. As the Witness, you do not have to become involved in the emotion at all. Let the character do all the work.

The image will vent your pain until it runs out of e-motion. At this stage, you will find it quite easy to bring your focus inward toward the observant aspect of your consciousness. Just as a mirror has no attachment to what it reflects, your Witnessing Self has no attachment to the character. As you watch the character expressing your emotions, they will be transformed. The mind wants to make this complicated so that it feels challenged, but it is really quite simple.

The Mind Wants You to Act Out the Image

As long as Tony remained identified with the image, he acted just like Rex the dog. He made a fuss about not wanting to be wrong and bad, while trying to prove that he was right and good. Every time Tony thought he had done something wrong, he would throw things in the air and go to his house to pout, emulating what Rex the dog did in his image. Tony reacted to stress in this manner long before he ever discovered his image of Rex the dog. When we apply The Witnessing Technique, the images that appear in the mind symbolically represent not only our pain, but also how we act out energetically or physically while we are under stress.

Had Tony been able to detach from the programming and identify with his Witnessing Self, he would have been able to *dis-identify* from the pain and the juvenile behavior his programming forced him to act out. He also would have recognized that he was not bad, and he had no need to try to prove his innocence. Being wrong and bad were only programmed ideas in his mind.

The point of this exercise is to observe that:
- *You are not the emotion—you are not the image—you are not the one in pain.*
- **You** are the **Witness** of these things.

If you can see the image, you are watching a symbolic projection of the mind's programming. The mind cannot watch itself. Who is the watcher? The watcher is Pure Consciousness. Once you identify with your *Witnessing Self,* you will be free from the ego's torment.

The Programming Will Always Be There in Your Mind

Programming is much like a record engraved with a voice. As stress occurs, the play button on your mental recording is pressed, and the voice on the soundtrack tells you how to react. You follow along, even if this advice has led you astray time and time again. When we identify with the mind, we are a slave to the recording. We cannot effectively alter this recording, (as much as the ego enjoys watching us try), but we can rise above it so that we are not controlled by it any longer.

Identify with Your Witnessing Self

Some people find their symbolism and stop there. They watch the image vent their emotions, but neglect to go to the next step, which is: **IDENTIFYING** WITH THE WITNESSING SELF.

Please understand that *you **are*** the neutral observer. *You are **not** the one in pain.* Your ego is the one in pain.

If you identify with the ego, you see the pain as your own. Identify instead with your *Witnessing Self,* and the pain will suddenly have nothing to do with you. *Embracing your identity as the witness is the key to rising above the programming once and for all.*

Positive Characters

Occasionally a positive character will emerge, such as a superhero ready to kill all the bad guys and sweep the love of his life off her feet. These positive characters must be observed as well, because they also represent programming in the mind.

Even though some of the programming makes us feel good, as long as we rely on it, we are involving ourselves with all the programming. If you choose the heroic programming, you are also choosing the villain programming. We cannot pick and choose, because it is all in the mind. We must observe everything the mind contains without becoming identified with it. Even a positive character will not be as empowering as choosing to identify with the pure, positive, playful energy of your source.

Choreographing

If you find yourself wanting to choreograph the character, it is a sure sign that your mind is fighting for control and that your Witnessing Self is no longer dominant. Even if you change the character into a more acceptable image, you will only become more enmeshed with the mind as you struggle to superimpose the new improved image over the old programming. Choreographing or changing the image will not bring about a neutral perspective. Without becoming a neutral witness to the image, you will remain trapped in the limited and often infantile behavioral range of the ego.

Choices

From the wise perspective of the *Witnessing Self*, you will be able to make a clear choice not to act on your mind's misguided suggestions. Eventually, your Soul Essence; which is your authentic self, will regain mastery over your life and all destructive behavior will cease.

> *When we are hypnotized by the mind, we become lost in its reflections. Think of your awareness as a mirror, and watch the reflections, but remain unattached. Know yourself always as the watcher.*

Because this is an entirely new way of living and responding, it is important to give yourself extra support throughout the day by recognizing when the mind is gaining strength and developing steam to push you toward its own agenda. To help make you more aware, we'll take a deeper look into the subtle control tactics the mind applies in order to keep us under its hypnotic spell.

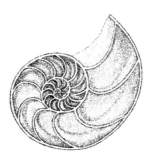

CHAPTER 3

Mental Energy

Introduction

Learning More about the Mind

THE PROGRAMMING THAT IS ETCHED INTO OUR MEMORY is so familiar to us that most of the time we don't even realize that it determines nearly everything we do. Once the subtle tactics of the mind are revealed, it will be easier to remain alert to its strategies and rise above the limitations and patterns by which we habitually live.

The mind itself is not the problem. It is our *identification* with the mind and its programming which presents our greatest challenges. When we perceive reality through the limited dualistic system of the mind, we become a puppet to its self-destructive ideas, which allows its negative perspective to determine our thoughts, beliefs, ideas, assumptions, emotions, and actions for us.

The more we rely on the mind, the less intelligent we become. Galileo, Copernicus, Kepler, Newton, Tesla, and Einstein all confess that their greatest discoveries occurred due to an *inner knowing* which was incongruent with the mind's limited boundaries and knowledge.

To experience a superior quality of intelligence, we must choose to be pioneers and enter a realm of clarity beyond the mind where greater wisdom and insight exist. Only then are we able to align with the true genius of our source.

The Mind's Limited View of Reality

According to the mind's limited perception of reality, humans are separate from Pure Consciousness. This statement is equivalent to saying that a light bulb is separate from the electric power source which provides the energy to create light.

Similar to a light bulb, without our source we have no power at all. When we blindly accept the mind's idea that humans are only physical matter, limited to their bodies and minds, we literally lose 98% of our power. In fact, the very idea of being separate is the root of ALL fear and powerlessness within humanity. Fear and powerlessness create the need for an ego. The *ego* forms a personality which emphasizes investing in a **purely physical** or **materialistic** *idea of power.*

Once we believe we are separate from our source, we feel the need to validate our existence. We do this by proving our worth through attaining power or importance in the physical world. The more ego centered an individual is, the more attached he will be to impressing, dominating, destroying, possessing, controlling, or being victorious over others in order to feel safe or adequate within society.

In extreme cases, the ego creates a desire for supremacy and the inclination to gain power over others through the use of force. The resulting violence and intimidation instigate wars, which are always a battle for power and control. Knives, guns, militaries, nuclear weapons, and terrorist organizations are all tools the ego uses to feel safe. According to the ego, we must rely on our physical force and mental cunningness to outsmart the enemy and get what we want. The ego is simply a defensive mechanism that is constantly fighting to gain more power over others in order to avoid the fear or humiliation of feeling inconsequential.

As you align with the higher power of Pure Consciousness, any feelings of inadequacy, as well as any fear of life or others, will disappear, and the desire to impress, conquer, or control will appear foolish. When you understand your source, you will know a power which extends far beyond your physical body. In fact, the energy that flows through you is considerably more potent than all nuclear weapons on the planet combined. Instead of being destructive, however, it is creative. The mind can hide this truth from you, but it cannot take it away.

Once you rise above the ego and view reality *free* from the mind's distorted version, you will know that you are not separate from the greatest power in Existence—you are part of it.

Everything is Vibration

It will be easier to see through the patterns that the mind applies by viewing life *vibrationally*.

The mind sees physical reality as solid, even though science has proven again and again that everything is made up of vibrating particles of energy. In actuality, nothing is solid. The lower vibrations simply appear solid to the average human eye. The higher or faster energy vibrates, the more open it is to the creative flow of Pure Consciousness. The slower the vibration, the less conscious it will be. With less consciousness, comes less power.

For example, a rock will hold less consciousness and less energy than a plant. A plant has more Life Force, so it has more vibrational power, freedom, and ability to grow. An animal will have more consciousness than a plant and, therefore, more vibrational energy, which provides greater power, freedom, and ability to evolve. Humans hold more consciousness than animals, and as a result, they have more vibrational power, freedom, and opportunity to transform.

Vibration

The On and Off Switch to Our Source

When a light switch is on, electricity can flow through the circuits to reach the bulb and illuminate it. When a light switch is off, an open circuit for the electric current does not exist. As humans we have an on and off switch to our electric current or Life Force as well. Our on and off switch is determined by the quality of our vibration. When our vibration is high, we are open to Pure Consciousness. When our vibration is low, we become more dense or closed.

What slows our vibration down the most is the ego and the attachments it forms, which cause emotional trauma. Pain, negativity, and unawareness lead to lower levels of consciousness. To stand apart from these negative influences, we'll examine how our thoughts, emotions, beliefs, and actions affect our vibration.

Thoughts and Emotions are Units of Energy

Thoughts are energy. Emotions are energy. Our own vibrational field is a compilation of the *quality* and *quantity* of the energy we radiate. If we wanted to measure the energetic units of thoughts and emotions, we could put a numerical quality to them similar to the list below. Although this list is not numerically accurate according to each individual at any moment in time, it gives a basic indication of the quality and quantity equated with specific fields of energetic output.

-indicates a deficit of energy
+ indicates a substantiation of energy

SPIRITUAL UNITS OF ENERGY

Unconsciousness −1000	Awareness +100,000

EMOTIONAL UNITS OF ENERGY

Shame −100	Self Love +1000
Guilt −90	Inner Peace +900
Hopelessness −80	Inner Joy +800
Sadness −70	Self-Acceptance +700
Fear −60	Compassion +600
Longing −50	Creativity +500
Anger −40	Courage +400

MENTAL UNITS OF ENERGY

Disappointment −90	Gratitude +900
Doubt −80	Understanding +800
Worry −70	Trust +700
Blame −60	Responsibility +600
Revenge −50	Detachment +500
Envy −40	Indifference +400

Scoring on the Energetic Scale

A high vibrational person will have a tremendously high score of quality energy, overflowing with Life Force, wanting to share their happiness and love with others. A low vibrational person will have a deficiency of energy and be much like a black hole in outer space—insatiable and empty, sucking energy from everyone who comes near them.

These opposite vibrations will attract opposite experiences due to the vibrational quality of the energy field that is being radiated. Similarly, you may experience a different reaction to someone who is very loving as opposed to someone who is very critical or depressed.

One person who has chosen to focus on hopelessness and fear, who thinks constantly of what a disappointment they are and how they blame their childhood for it, may deplete their Life Force as much as −290 on the energetic scale within a few minutes. As they remain focused on their negativity, they diminish not only their own energy field further, but also the energy field of anyone around them who is not connected to his own power source. Lethargy, depression and a feeling of being scattered are often the result.

A vibration of −290 units of energy will also be radiating and attracting more disappointment and desire to blame, as well as more fear and hopelessness. The lower an individual's vibration drops, the more it damages health, quality of intelligence, and ability to experience harmony with others. Every added second of negative focus will increase the negative units of energy they radiate. Within a few minutes, this person could reach a new low of −450 units of energy, which may energetically repulse anyone who comes near them. A lower vibration renders us more unconscious, so it is often difficult for a despondent person to understand that it is within their own power to transform their energy and become a higher vibration.

On the other hand, an individual who has risen above the ego and discovered an authentic love for life, may have an energetic score of +3800 units of energy. This person will feel deep gratitude and lives each moment in celebration, excited to apply her own creative Life Force, constantly manifesting more of what brings her joy. As an added bonus, her vibration will attract more experiences that will enhance her love for life, and her vibration will continue to rise. These types of individuals will act as an uplifting force to anyone who comes near them. Their presence alone exudes a tremendously beneficial power. Therefore, *the greatest contribution any of us can make is to* **raise our own vibration.**

Do Thoughts and Emotions Create Our Reality?

As you raise your level of awareness, you will begin to notice that thoughts and emotions directly affect your vibration. Your vibration attracts circumstances and people to you who match the level of consciousness you radiate. *Everything is energy which vibrates and aligns according to vibrational similarities.*

Even the thought of *not* wanting something will be sending out a vibration that attracts what you do not want. Have you ever noticed that when you flick a bug away, it will run right back in your direction each time? When we have an aversion (negative thought) or an interest (positive thought) coupled with a potent emotion, the energy acts as an attractor beam, drawing to us the balance of our vibration. It does not matter if these thoughts and emotions are negative or positive. The attractor beam radiates outward, drawing in the balance of that energy. *To raise our vibration and get what we want, we must learn to remove our focus from what we do not want and place it on what we do want.*

What We Send Out Returns to Us

You cannot battle against something and expect to be victorious. Those who fight for peace with angry protesting are unknowingly adding to the vibration of war. On the other hand, focusing on a creative solution that stimulates love, harmony, and compassion will add to peace.

Those who condemn their leaders, parents, partners, children, friends, business associates, and teachers are unknowingly attracting behavior from these people that will lead to more disappointment. Those who appreciate others attract more harmony in their relationships.

If you focus on something that disturbs you, you are attracting it into your life. If you focus on something that delights you, you are attracting it into your life. The best use we can make of our mental energy is to remain focused on solutions and thoughts that align with our positive intentions. A high vibrational being will do this instinctively, because this person's energy is always creative.

Every Thought Creates a Destination

Imagine each thought as a destination, and every second you think of that thought, you are traveling one mile in that direction.

One second of thought = One "energetic" mile toward that destination.

The longer your mind remains focused on one specific thought, the closer you are coming to that destination. It does not matter if the thought is negative or positive; you will travel closer to its destination each second.

If the thought upon which you are most focused happens to be negative or painful, then a trauma zone filled with conflict might be your destination. If the trauma zone is 120 "energetic" miles away, every second you think your destructive thought, you are getting one mile closer to conflict. After two minutes of destructive thinking, you will arrive at your painful destination and step into a reality already **created by you with your very own mental energy.**

The nature of your thoughts will deliver you into a set of circumstances that represent each moment spent on your thinking journey.

Once you arrive at your destructive destination, you are likely to experience even more pain, which creates more intense thoughts and emotions. These new thoughts may be taking you toward a destination of personal injury. If these thoughts ignite extreme anger, your next destination will be closer, and it will take less time to arrive.

*The **thought** creates the **destination,** and the **emotion** determines the **distance** to that destination.*

The intensity of the emotion behind the thought shortens the distance toward your destination. Now that your anger has intensified, your personal injury zone may only be 60 "energetic" miles away, so it will only take you one minute of rageful thinking to arrive there.

This equation applies to positive thoughts as well. If you have thoughts of appreciation, then your destination will be a reward zone. Every second you focus on gratitude, you come one mile closer to your destination. If you feel great passionate love for life as you look around in appreciation, your reward zone may be as close as ten "energetic" miles from where you are right now, which will only take ten seconds of joyful thinking.

How to Use the Mind

The best use you can make of the mind is to:

1) Know what you want.

2 Be clear about how that would make you feel.

3) Vibrate that feeling by imagining you are already living that reality.

The mind does not know the difference between real or imagined. Therefore, whatever you vibrate, even if it is only the balance of your happy imagination, your mind will assume it to be real. If you could imagine or visualize your happiest life and then act as though you are already living the balance of that new reality, everything would align with these new ideas very quickly.

Applying this recipe as often as possible will be beneficial. However, we must also consider the stress factor in life.

The Stress Factor

Not only do positive thoughts and emotions create positive experiences, they also act as buffers, moment by moment canceling out the balance of your core fears and mental programming. The trouble arises when you are under stress. Then your positive thoughts and emotions are not as easily generated, and your core fears are given the ability to gain the momentum they would not usually gain while you were feeling strong and happy.

Positive thoughts and emotions certainly uplift us and add to our joy. Yet, generating thoughts and emotions which counteract the effect of our mental programming or ego personality, will only take us so far in life. If you want to live free from the struggle and pain your programming attracts, you must rise above the mental programming which causes pain altogether. At that moment you will no longer be vibrationally susceptible to the stress factor.

Once you rise above the programming and begin to identify with your Soul Essence, you will vibrate ecstatic energy predominantly, and your thoughts and emotions will continue to create rewarding destinations. You will still be able to use the mind, but the mind will no longer be able to use you.

The Effects of Ego and Programming

The ego is innately problem oriented, always wanting to defend against its fears, which makes it prone to creating lack. On the other hand, your inner being, or Pure Consciousness, is overflowing with so much pure, positive, creative energy, that it is capable of effortlessly manifesting an abundance of everything you want.

If you find yourself without enough health, wealth, love, joy, or opportunity, the mind will come in and frighten you by immediately focusing on the problem—which lowers your vibration and creates a destination where you will be experiencing more lack. If you can rise above the mind during moments of stress, you will align with the abundant power of your source. Consequently, your circumstances will transform rapidly. What do you think pure, positive, creative energy would do in a situation of lack? It certainly would not consult a fearful, negative mind for advice. It would dive right into the joy of creating abundantly with absolute confidence, knowing its success is guaranteed.

If you are vibrating exhaustion from working hard at a job you hate just so you can pay the bills, you will be generating thoughts and emotions which form a destination where you can expect to experience more hard work that needs to be done, more exhaustion, and more bills to pay. As you continue to stimulate defeating emotions, you draw to you more depleting destinations.

When you rise above the fear and worry of the mind, you enter a vibrational frequency that stimulates thoughts and emotions of joy, ease, abundance, and support. These thoughts and emotions create a destination where you can experience a natural influx of joy, ease, abundance, and support.

The actions you take, how hard you work, the amount of talent you have, how much time you spend, and how much help you have, will not affect your reality as much as your vibration. When you rise above the mind, you tap into the infinite flow of pure, positive, creative Life Force (the highest vibration available), and everything that aligns with your idea of bliss will begin to flow immediately toward you.

Remember: you are pure, positive, creative energy. Once you align with this truth, all of the situations your fearful programming created for you will transform. You are not the past, and you are not your pain. You are pure, positive, creative energy that can do anything, be anything, and create anything. That is the real you. You have infinite power to transform your life and thrive as the person you have always dreamed of being, just by rising above the limited ideas in your mind that form unwanted vibrations.

Core Fears and Programmed Beliefs

Even when you are not focused on a specific thought or emotion, you continue to radiate a vibration. This vibration will be generated by your core fears and programmed beliefs. Although our conscious thoughts and emotions contribute to the totality of our vibration and continually create new destinations for us, our core fears and programmed beliefs affect our energy field more consistently.

Our core fears form our personality—our way of thinking, feeling, acting, and reacting to life. A strong, mentally-generated positive thought will only take us as far as the ego or mental programming will allow.

Many people project positive thoughts and positive emotions, yet they still find themselves creating circumstances that do not match up with what they want. No matter how mentally and emotionally positive we are, we must rise above the ego in order to bypass the influence our programming has on our vibrational template. Once we become the *witness* to our core fears and mental programming, we will no longer take the pain that ego generates seriously, and we will be more likely to create experiences that align more harmoniously and immediately with our conscious intentions.

For a thorough understanding of how to influence the totality of our vibration, we must recognize how these factors impact our lives. With greater clarity, we begin to comprehend how we get what we get.

Common Effect of the Core Fear

Imagine a woman who suffers from the *core fear* of being *unworthy of love*. Her entire personality has been formed in defense of this fear. Even if this woman constantly thinks positive thoughts, her core fear will surface throughout the day with very little provocation.

This woman may have recently spent two weeks enjoying a love-filled honeymoon, but her core fear of being unworthy of love will still stimulate concern that she could be rejected, abandoned, or separated from her lover in some way. These thoughts will pop into her mind whenever she is feeling stress, creating doubt and negativity in her perfect love life.

Her fears might be accentuated on the plane ride home from her honeymoon when she notices how tight her skirt has become from gaining five pounds on the trip. If she happens to notice a very beautiful and slender flight attendant walking by, it will be enough for her to react defensively to her core fear of being unworthy of love. When the beautiful flight attendant approaches her row of seats, this woman will monitor her husband and react negatively to any positive attention he gives the flight attendant.

Her husband's attention to the other woman will bring up her deepest pain, which is her fear of being unworthy of love. No matter how much she focuses her thoughts and emotions toward those things that make her feel loved, the ego's negative perspective of self will continue to ignite her fears.

Another detrimental aspect of the ego is its power to block our ability to understand that our pain is self-generated. Without the core fear of being unworthy of love, this woman would not experience any pain if her husband smiled at another beautiful woman, because she would feel secure within herself. The ego is always ready to give our power away and blame the pain it generates on some outside circumstance or person. Instead of taking responsibility for our pain, (which would give us the power to eliminate it), the ego will assume it is up to others to live according to our rules and expectations, so that we can avoid our fears. This mind-set leads to disappointment.

The wife, who identifies herself with the core fear of being unworthy of love, will leave it up to her husband to make her feel loved and wanted. According to her ego, it is his responsibility as her partner. She will also feel validated in restricting and manipulating her husband in an attempt to make sure he is doing everything right in accordance with what she believes will make her feel loved and wanted in a marriage. This possessive energy will restrict the husband to such a degree that he will eventually feel unhappy with the union and decide to leave, or he will become aloof to the wife's constant need for singular attention and reassurance that she is indeed the only one he loves and wants. Her core fears will attract to her the abandonment she fears.

Once we take responsibility for rising above our core fears, we begin to experience the quality of love and happiness we deserve in life. In order to rise above the ego, we must stand apart from the mind and remain aloof or detach from the fears it imposes on us.

Common Effects of Programmed Beliefs

Our programmed beliefs are also more influential to our vibration than our conscious thoughts and emotions. We can use the example of a man who has just turned forty and finds himself thirty pounds overweight with wrinkles forming and hair falling out. If this man begins right away to focus on youth, vitality, and a healthy head of hair, his thoughts and desires will begin to change his vibration and create a destination where he will experience more vitality, youth, and the re-growth of hair on his head.

His positively focused thoughts and emotions will bring him closer to a more youthful destination every second, until these new ideas disturb the programmed beliefs he holds, which contradict his goals. In his deeper belief system, his mind may have equated aging with overweight, unappealing, bald men. As he vibrates the balance of his beliefs, he will reach a threshold that his consciously generated, positive thoughts and intentions cannot easily break through. This programming is so ingrained in him that it carries more vibrational power and *keeps his unconscious thoughts* focused in the direction of further aging, even though he consciously wants to reach a destination of greater youth.

Most of our concrete ideas about reality have been held in our belief systems since we were children. This man may have listened to an aging grandfather complain about no longer receiving attention from women, and mistakenly believed that to be the plight of all aging men. However, these self-destructive beliefs will not be the only negative programming that his personality holds about aging. He could superimpose positive thoughts over his negative belief system for the rest of his life, as he struggles to keep the balance of his negativity about physical reality at bay. Alternatively, he could rise above his mental programming, align with Pure Consciousness, and vibrate far above and beyond the reach of any of his programmed beliefs. In this manner, he will reach the success he desires, by recreating his youthful vitality.

Vibrating Above

Core Fears and Mental Programming

From the Witnessing perspective, you step into your true magnificence, completely detached from the programmed ideas you hold about what is good, bad, right, wrong, negative, positive, fat, skinny, young, old, etc.

Those who have learned to identify with Pure Consciousness, radiate a vibration which reflects Source Energy. Those who identify with the mind and their ego personality, radiate a vibration that reflects their core fears and programmed beliefs.

As you remain in the vibration of your source, your reality will not only align with the pure, positive, playful energy of Pure Consciousness, you will also experience transformation and rejuvenation without struggle.

While it is true that our conscious thoughts and emotions vibrate and magnetically attract to us a destination of their likeness, we have many deeper and more penetrating ideas about reality that are always vibrating whether we are aware of them or not. You will no longer be troubled by your ego or mental programming once you rise above the mind and vibrate in alignment with Pure Consciousness.

As you apply The Witnessing Technique, you will learn to stand apart from the ego by identifying with the aspect of your consciousness that simply *observes* your fears and beliefs as a neutral bystander. Once this shift occurs, your vibration will align with Pure Consciousness quite naturally.

The following chapter outlines specific tactics the mind employs in order to dominate our response to life and keep us tethered to our core fears and programmed beliefs.

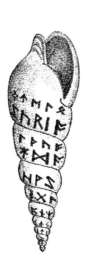

CHAPTER 4

Mind Tricks

Prejudice

ONE PERSON MAY BE DISTURBED BY A CERTAIN RACE OR RELIGION while another is inspired. These perspectives are only due to what we have been programmed to believe regarding what is good, bad, right, and wrong. When we align with the neutral energy of Pure Consciousness, we realize there are no good or bad people. We all flow with the neutral energy of Pure Consciousness, which is where the saying, "We are all created equal," originated. It is only the ego, not the Soul Essence, that feels driven toward judgments and actions that oppose love or Divinity.

Labeling people as good or bad creates a tremendous depletion of vital Life Force. Once you become disinterested in judgments and categorizations, your level of energy and intelligence will rise significantly, and your ability to love and accept yourself and others will expand.

Gossip

Gossip is usually based on who we think is bad and who we think is good, who we think is right and who we think is wrong, who made us happy and who has made us sad. Gossip is one of the fastest ways to engage the ego, rendering us more deeply entrenched in negative programming.

When we stop categorizing and criticizing others, we stop categorizing and criticizing ourselves, because the critical part of the mind loses momentum. Recognize the strong hold the ego has over you when it inspires you to gossip, and choose not to indulge. Simply watch the thoughts, and soon they will pass. You will be a little freer from the programming each time you practice being the *neutral witness* of your urge to gossip.

The Mind is a Commentator

The mind wants to turn everything it views into words. It is a generator of thoughts, needing to comment on everything. If you come across an unusually pleasant scene, the mind may say, "This is so beautiful." These words limit the whole experience, because words themselves are very limiting. Thoughts and words diminish the expansive reality of life. The mind always tries to turn a vast experience into a small one so that it feels in control.

Play this game: Sit in front of an ocean or a forest and simply experience *being* with nature. Allow the experience to touch you without thinking. Open to the majesty and beauty that surround you. If you allow the experience in without words, you will feel a vastness that is intangible and empowering. Afterwards, you will feel energized and uplifted.

Next, allow your mind to comment on everything you notice about the scene. Stay in your mind, and *think* about how much you like it. Then sense your energy. You will feel as though you are missing something great. The expansive magic of Existence can not be pressed into words. It can only be felt when you are in the moment, allowing yourself to be aware of what is present without the mind's comments.

To strengthen your connection with Pure Consciousness, begin experiencing the beauty or Divinity of life, instead of pressing it into words. When you experience life without words, you will be far more fulfilled, and the unlimited power and potential of Existence will begin to penetrate your being.

Perspective

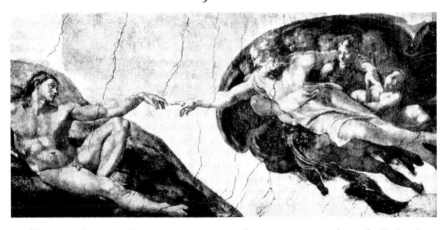

The mind can only see a tiny aspect of any greater truth, and all absolute truths contain contradiction. A *near-sighted* gentleman touring the Sistine Chapel, may be admiring Michelangelo's Fresco, *The Creation of Adam*, (shown above) having only the visual capacity to make out the finger of God in the painting. A *far-sighted* gentleman viewing the same masterpiece, might be able to capture the entire scene of God reaching out to

Man, but God's finger may appear blurry and inconsequential to him on the whole. Both gentlemen will be looking at the same work of art, but what they are capable of seeing is very different. These two individuals will argue over what the fresco contains and both of them will be right, according to their own tiny perspectives.

If a Michelangelo connoisseur with perfect vision were to join the discussion, he may agree with the first fellow and be able to admire the beauty of God's finger. He will also be able to marvel at the image of God and Man reaching out to one another. His main focus, however, may be on the entire chapel. Because his perspective is vast, he will comprehend the near-sighted and far-sighted point of views, understanding they are both correct according to their own narrow perspectives.

The same situation applies to all disagreements between people. Everyone clings to the aspect of truth they are capable of seeing with their personal abilities. Those who are more identified with their mind and ego will have the most limited perception of the truth, and those identified with Pure Consciousness, will be aware of the bigger picture.

When we rise above the mind, we understand a reality that is not only physical, but energetic; not learned, but experienced; not finite, but infinite. Those stuck in the mind will fight for their limitations as if other people's perspectives threaten their very existence.

How do you teach a blind man to behold light? You give him eyes that can see. Unless you rise above the mind, you will never be able to comprehend the power and magnificence of Pure Consciousness. As the *witness*, you enter a world where a more expansive reality exists. In this greater reality, you will find it easier to understand and maintain harmony with fellow citizens.

The Mind is a Pendulum

The mind can complain and criticize. It can praise and give compliments. It cannot, however, remain choiceless. It must choose one side, and once it does, the choice it has made is bound to change within a short span of time. Lovers can adore each other in the morning, but by the afternoon their minds will become focused on the less than lovable qualities about each other. The mind will be happy or sad, content or discontent, infatuated or fed up. Like a pendulum, it is constantly swinging back and forth all day long. This is simply the nature of the mind.

When the mind moves to one extreme, it builds momentum to swing all the way to the other extreme. It is impossible to choose only one side, just as it is impossible to say, "I will only inhale from now on, I will no longer exhale." The two go together. The negative and positive poles of the mind make up one unit. They rely on each other. Instructing someone to think positively and assuring them that only good things will follow, is much like saying, "Just keep on inhaling. Do not exhale, and all good things will come to pass."

The idea of being able to create what we want with positive thought is very exciting. People will feel uplifted, empowered, and optimistic for a few hours or days as they apply their positive thoughts to everything in their life. Then suddenly, for no apparent reason, the mind takes its natural pendulum swing and fear, negativity, doubt, anger, shame, anxiety, and sadness will follow. The higher the positive swing, the lower the negative swing will feel.

Average humans will beat themselves up and think they have done something wrong, because they can not remain positive enough to lose the extra weight, get the promotion, or stop smoking. Once this happens, they may give up hope, assuming they do not have what it takes to create what they want. However, their inability to remain positive is not their fault. The mind is a pendulum. It works much like gravity—what goes up must come down.

Without this unpleasant pendulum swing, we would not have as much incentive to rise above the mind and finally live free from the dualistic experience of life it offers us. The pendulum effect gives us yet another reason to align with the neutral, non-judgmental, unlimited, boundless, infinite, symbiotic aspect of our consciousness, which is free from the pendulum-swinging roller coaster of the mind.

If you want to **remain** positive, you must rise above the mind and identify with the neutral aspect of your being that already exists in a pure, positive reality, free from duality and attachments. Once you connect with your Soul Essence, your life will transform quickly, without struggling to project positive thoughts. This shift becomes permanent, as you learn to view life from the higher perspective of Pure Consciousness, rather than the limited dualistic mechanism of the mind, with all its attachments, rules, defeatisms, and judgments.

If it is fun for you to play with positive thoughts, do so. Visualize, fantasize, imagine, laugh, sing, dance, and enjoy. When you reach the pendulum swing, however, and find yourself back in the negative end of the mind, do not beat yourself up. Dive right into The Witnessing Technique and remain the neutral unattached observer of your programming as it tries to sabotage your reality with its negative ideas.

Eventually you will sense the negative thoughts as they begin to build, and you will be able to remain detached, *no longer identifying with the pain and fear in the mind.* As the witness, you will maintain a very high vibration, even when the mind is negative, thereby, allowing greater potential to continually create uplifting destinations and rewarding experiences.

Desire

What we believe we desire and what we truly need are often two different things. The mind itself is what deludes us by projecting blame or longing outside of the self. We may want to hurt someone when we are angry or possess someone when we are infatuated, but these are mental placebos that cover up a deeper need.

For example, the husband with compulsive rage may project his anger onto his wife and desire to kill her, believing his anger will be extinguished along with his wife. Even if he kills her, the rage will survive. His true need is to achieve inner peace, not to kill his wife. However, the mind will project such a strong image of blame onto the wife, that the husband will be unable to make the separation and recognize his real need.

Even in the case of infatuation, ego is responsible. The desire to possess a specific person may be covering up a deep fear of being empty, alone, or unloved. The real need is to rise above the inner emptiness, so that even when the individual is single, they will feel whole and happy about life.

In another instance, a person who believes he desires alcohol may be covering up a deeper need to accept himself and have confidence around others. Alcohol may feel like an avenue of escape from anxiety or judgments, but the inner critic will only gain strength each time the alcohol is taken, and more alcohol will be desired. If the person were to identify and work on his real need, which is to accept the self, his desire for alcohol would diminish.

Whenever you have a strong desire, look more deeply and find the true need beneath it. Then move toward fulfilling the true need. You will create a profound shift into higher levels of awareness where the mind has less control over your behavior.

Attachment

Once the mind has separated us from Pure Consciousness, our programming will convince us that happiness, safety, and stability are all dependent on the physical world. We form attachments and fears based on these ideas. The more we rely on the outer world for our feelings of safety, security, happiness, and love, the more attachments we form. Our personality, or the way we want to be seen, (in order to feel safe) becomes our greatest attachment of all. Yet the image or identity we create is merely a façade to hide our core fears from ourselves and others.

1) The person with a **core fear of being bad** may become attached to building an image which makes them appear noble, wise, kind, pure, modest, moderate, self-disciplined, just, and good, so they can be seen as innocent, chaste or saint-like in the eyes of others. To achieve this, they often develop into the incessant do-gooder, the hardest worker, the minimalist, the religious fanatic, the law enforcer, the charity worker, the environmentalist, and other similar careers. Without the pretense of the image they desire, they feel insecure and afraid that others will perceive them as bad, evil, deviant, or corrupt. If they fail to reach the image they seek, they invest their energies in pointing out all the (real or imagined) bad or deviant qualities in others. They may take on the role of the tattle-tailing child, the righteous reformer, the abrasive corrector, the opinionated oppressor, the rigid moralizer, the punitive judge, the unforgiving punisher, the intolerant critic, the rationalizing evil-doer, the impatient condemner, the secret deviant, or the callous dogmatic. The ego casts them in these roles in order to take their focus away from their own feared flaws and deviances.

2) The person with a **core fear of being unworthy of love** may become attached to building an image where they believe they will be seen as the most loved and wanted within society. To achieve this, they often

focus their attention on their appearance, sexuality, or communicative abilities by becoming the helpful child, the flirt, the model, the actor, the people pleaser, the flatterer, the selfless caregiver, the thoughtful angel, the healer, the hostess, the good friend, or the charity volunteer, among others. Without the pretense of a lovable image, they turn hopeless and become emotionally unstable, desperate, and frightened that no one will ever love them. According to their ego, being single or unattached proves they are unwanted and unworthy of love. If they are unable to reach the image they desire, they may take on the role of the victim, the martyr, the eternal sufferer, the predator, the nymphomaniac, the possessive partner, the obsessed, the brokenhearted, the guilt-instilling manipulator, the unsolicited advice giver, the psychic, the worrier, the invasive smotherer, the weeper, the whiner, the drama queen or king, the emotional eater, the remuneration seeker, or the hypochondriac. The ego casts them in these roles in order to elicit love, affection, and neediness from others, so they can escape their fear of being unloved and unwanted.

3) The person with the **core fear of being unimportant** will become attached to forming an image where they will appear superior to others. To achieve the power and status they desire, they often focus their energy toward gaining material proof that they are the best. They strive to become millionaires in their twenties, politicians, professional athletes, celebrities, or powerful and important business executives, and other high profile personalities. They may develop into the attention seeking child, the aggressive self-promoter, the effective planner, the overachiever, the charismatic flirt, the self-improvement guru, the motivator, the show off, the cunning competitor, the vigilant opportunist, the industrious worker, the image conscious projector, the manipulative charmer, the political candidate, or the failure phobic. Without the pretense of an important image, they become angry and dangerously vengeful toward those who appear superior to them. If they fail to reach the success they desire, they focus their intense energy

on manufacturing an impressive image. In their quest, they may take on the role of the jealous partner, the psychopathic liar, the fake-it-till-you-make-it phony, the exploiter, the distinguished con artist, the scheming saboteur, the divisive criminal, the vengeful attacker, the pot shot comic, or the narcissistic sociopath. The ego casts them in these roles in an attempt to make a mark in society, and escape their fear of not being important enough.

4) The person with the **core fear of having no purpose or significance** in life will become attached to forming an image in which they appear to be invaluable, special, unique, or extraordinary. To achieve this they want to be original and bigger than life. They often develop into self-appointed spiritual leaders, artists, musicians, poets, or entrepreneurs in some flamboyant field. To achieve an intense feeling of having purpose, they want the world to validate and support them emotionally. In an attempt to elicit the support they seek, they may convert to being the moody child, the super-sensitive acquaintance, the outspoken intuitive, the fickle lover, the deep feeler, or the attention-starved expresser. Without the pretense of having a very special image, they turn exceedingly negative, blameful, depressed, or suicidal, often taking on the role of the temperamental blamer, the brooding sulker, the depressed addict, the demanding malcontent, the difficult relative, the guilt-instilling complainer, the self-absorbed narcissist, the aloof mutant, the self-loathing dark cloud, the perpetual pessimist, the inappropriate truth teller, or the stuck-in-the-pain-of-the-past victim. The ego casts these people in roles where they can feel some sense of self, (even if it is a painful identification) so they can escape their fear of having no purpose.

5) The person with the **core fear of being unable to apply their own personal power,** may become attached to having extreme levels of privacy or alone time in order to avoid their fear of being overpowered. To achieve this they often recede within themselves and develop into the

shy child, the deep thinker, the nervous observer, the secretive inno-
vator, the mysterious recluse, the busy worker, the studious researcher,
the independent genius, the artful dodger, the self-sustaining expert,
the private acquaintance, or the unsociable colleague. Without the
solitude and free time they desire to pursue their passions in the safety
of their own presence, they may disappear from society altogether or
turn to harsher means of keeping others away. To achieve this they
may take on the role of the cynical bystander, the agitated friend, the
antagonizing debater, the bridge-burner, the disappearing artist, the
unaccommodating acquaintance, the absent-minded professor, or the
detached schizophrenic. The ego casts them in these roles in order to
create alone space where they feel safe to apply their power and escape
their fear of being incapacitated or dishonored by others.

6) The person with the **core fear of being unsafe or insecure** on their
own may become attached to finding group support, a committed-
trustworthy partner, growing investments, and family collaboration in
order to feel safe. To achieve this they often develop into the security-
seeking child, the engaging acquaintance, the seductive romantic, the
committed lobbyist, the political support leader, the church group
coordinator, the team captain or coach, the methodical worker, the
action-oriented parent, the involved neighbor, the professional
student, the teacher, the group organizer, the community representative, the politician, the institute founder, the union representative, the
group travel coordinator, the fund raiser, or the charity founder. If they
fail to rally the support systems they believe they need in order to feel
safe, secure, and supported by others, they can easily develop panic
attacks or high levels of anxiety that consume their lives. This causes
passive-aggressive behavior meant to threaten others into supporting
them. They may take on the role of the betraying partner, the overwhelmed parent, the anxiety-ridden seducer, the clingingly dependent
ex-lover, the irrational betrayer, the promiscuous drifter, the scape-
goating conspirator, the night club hopper, the panicking masochist,

the unreliable pal, the untrustworthy business associate, or the forever tardy date. The ego casts them in these roles in order to elicit the unconditional support they desire so they can feel safe and secure.

7) The person with the **core fear of loss and deprivation** may become attached to extreme levels of stimulation, such as constant companionship, attention, fame, glamour, wealth, prestige, and power. To achieve their goal, they often develop into the extroverted child, the variety-seeking enthusiast, the outgoing acquaintance, the cheerful adventurer, the energetic party thrower, the gregarious business associate, the talkative attention seeker, the shock jock, the talented comedian, the story teller, the constant entertainer, the ostentatious performer, or the dazzling dancer or musician. Without a grandiose or showy image, they may become manic, childish, and reckless; often turning toward drugs, sex, alcohol, food, sugar, shopping, gambling, travel, or risk taking in order to maintain high levels of stimulation. They may take the role of the forever occupied dilettante, the sensationalist, the dangerous pleasure pursuer, the hyperactive attention grabber, the uninhibited thrill seeker, the wasteful extravagant, the insatiable sadomasochist, the compulsive shoplifter, the manic depressant, the reckless infantile, the excessive addict, the greedy dissatisfied, the overdrawn gambler, or the tortured schizophrenic. The ego casts them in these roles in order to reach the level of stimulation they believe they need to feel fulfilled by life.

8) The person with the **core fear of being vulnerable to harm** may become attached to being in control of everything and everyone in their lives. To achieve this they often develop into the street-smart child, the strong-willed acquaintance, the super-determined persuader, the tenacious hero, the overly self-confident leader, the father figure, the decisive challenger, the strategic justice seeker, the forceful negotiator, the shrewd entrepreneur, the resolute, the bully, the intimidator, or the confrontationalist. Without the feeling of being in control, they can

turn ruthless, brutally dominating, and dictatorial, often taking on the role of the cruel and controlling boss, the egocentric date, the intimidating oppressor, the remorseless polygamist, the outlaw, the violent dictator, the heartless megalomaniac, the dominating tyrant, the murderous sociopath, or the destructive monster. The ego casts them in these roles in an attempt to gain control over others so they can finally feel safe within society.

9) The person with the **core fear of being disturbed** will often become attached to a certain avenue of escape or fantasy that they can rely on whenever they are faced with unpleasant situations. In an attempt to maintain harmony, they transform into whoever they think they need to be, in order to please the people they are currently with. They may develop into the gentle child, the peaceful pal, the easy-going parent, the mild-mannered friend, the patient partner, the graceful arbitrator, the healing presence, the supportive acquaintance, or the accommodating leader. If their self-diminishing plans to maintain harmony fail and they are still faced with painful realities, they may turn incoherent, aloof, non-responsive, completely shut down, or subservient to anyone who is upset, by becoming the compliant wimp, the dutiful parent, the selective communication receptor, the unresponsive mate, the silent punching bag, the shut-down lover, the vacant person, the catatonic robot, the unavailable family member, or the lost soul. The ego casts them in these roles in order to avoid the pain of their reality so they can feel safe.

Once the ego has cast us in these roles, we perfect them more each day without ever realizing that the image we project does not reflect our authentic self. By identifying with the neutral energy of Pure Consciousness, we can find a safe, fulfilling, stable experience of elation, which is independent of the personality we have built or the attachments to which we cling.

Infatuation

Another Dangerous Attachment

- If you *observe* an emotional experience and it *expands*, it is *real*.

- If you *observe* an emotional experience and it *disperses or changes under stress*, then it was only a projection of the *ego*.

If your partner falls in love with someone else and you are able to set them free while continuing to feel reverence for them, you know real love. You are aligned with the unattached, free-flowing bliss of Pure Consciousness. If your partner falls in love with someone else and you suddenly hate him or her, want to possess them more, wish them misery or blame them for your pain, your original feelings were only based in infatuation, attachment, or possessiveness—which are projections of the ego. *True love is a state of being.* Attachment and possessiveness are a construction of the mind.

Infatuation feels powerful because it involves extreme levels of desire. It is such a strong force that the mind can easily convince you that it is love. This has given love a bad name. *Love has never broken a single heart,* but possession, attachment, obsession, lust, and infatuation have the potential to break your heart and wound your pride each time.

Everything we become attached to in life will eventually fade. Lovers come and go, jobs come and go, friends come and go, fame comes and goes, life comes and goes, but Pure Consciousness always remains. The blissful energy of our source is timeless and eternal. *Pure Consciousness is the only thing upon which we can **always** rely.* Once you rise above attachments, you will know freedom for the first time.

Duality and Neutrality

Mind is built on duality, so we want to *step aside from duality* whenever possible. Our source is neutral, so we want to *align with neutrality* as much as possible. You must remain neutral to the programming in the mind in order to align with the tremendous energy of Pure Consciousness. Only in this neutral, unattached, unbiased state will you begin to experience the indescribable bliss that can only be found beyond the realms of the mind.

Pure Consciousness is always with us, always loving us, always supporting us, always blissful. When we finally become tired of reaching outside of ourselves for fulfillment in the material world, we are left with only one other place to go, which is within. And that is where the real treasures exist.

The following chapter will simplify the process of moving within and offer further guidance that will assist you in rising above the mind and elevating your level of consciousness more each day.

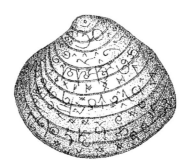

CHAPTER 5

Rising Above the Mind

Relativity

Everything is Relative—According to Vibration

WHEN EINSTEIN ANNOUNCED HIS THEORY OF RELATIVITY, the minds of many were disturbed. How can something as rigid and factual as time be relative they argued. According to Einstein, if a rocket leaves the planet traveling faster than the speed of light, a passenger aboard could travel for twenty-five years and return to earth as if no time had passed at all. Earthbound friends would have aged twenty-five years; but for the passenger, time stood still.

Einstein's discovery is invaluable when it comes to understanding consciousness. Time is an invention of the mind. In the realms of Pure Consciousness, time does not exist. Time and space help us live in a physical reality by giving us guidelines to work around, similar to setting up rules in the game of chess. Time is simply a boundary to which we agree. Therefore, it is relative.

In Einstein's example, moving faster than the speed of light would raise the traveler's vibration to such great heights that he would be unable to live within the boundaries of the mind where time exists. Without the constraints of the mind, he cannot age. Pure Consciousness is timeless and eternal.

When we align with the boundaries of the mind, we lower ourselves into a denser vibration, which absorbs our power. The purpose of this buffered reality is to protect us from our own fears, ideas, beliefs, thoughts, and emotions—which would instantly attract to us the content of our mind, if it were not for the safety valve of our cushioned existence. Physical reality could be named "Wielding Life Force 101," a course designed to help us understand how to apply our power while wearing a safety belt. Those who learn to stand apart from their thoughts and emotions by *witnessing* the mind, achieve mastery over their power and graduate beyond the thresholds of physical reality.

Einstein's theory established that age (or time) is determined by speed or vibration. The people existing on earth will age in accordance with the rotational speed of this planet, as well as the level of energy they are personally vibrating. On another planet that moved at twice the speed of earth, the beings present there would age at a slower rate, because the vibration would be higher. We may not have direct control over how fast our planet rotates, but we do have control over our own level of energy and the speed of our own personal vibration. The fastest way to raise our vibration (and our consciousness) is to stop identifying with the mind's boundaries (which are all relative) and open ourselves to Universal Energy instead.

Vibration Determines Behavior

When our vibration changes, our behavior changes. Similar to an ice cube that raises its vibration and transforms into warm mist, our vibration affects our behavior as well. Warm mist cannot act the same as an ice cube. All vibrational transformation changes behavior.

Raising our level of consciousness is the only way to effectively free ourselves from the past and the frozen habits mind forms. When we raise our vibration, our behavior aligns closer with Pure Consciousness, which is Pure Love or Divine Intelligence.

Do not waste time trying to impose restraints, rules, laws, morals, or beliefs in order to form new habits. That would be like trying to teach a block of ice how to act like warm mist without first changing its vibration. You would be asking the impossible, and the poor ice-cube would grow an inferiority complex and become more hopeless each time it failed.

The way we think, feel, act, and respond to life, ourselves, and others, all changes as we raise our vibration, simply because our vibration determines our level of consciousness, and our level of consciousness determines our behavior.

Raising Consciousness

Five basis areas lift the totality of our vibration and increase our level of consciousness. Listed here in order of importance, they are:

Spiritual

Emotional

Mental

Physical

Environmental

To obtain maximum benefits, it is helpful to focus our attention on raising our vibration in all five areas *daily*, placing most of our focus on our spiritual vibration, which is our awareness of the fact that we are Pure Consciousness. We are Universal Energy focused in a physical body.

Acceleration

Uplifting Spiritual Vibration

Awareness of Pure Consciousness (how to align with it or know ourselves through it) is the most significant shift anyone can make to raise their vibration. There are two very powerful methods of accomplishing this—The Witnessing Technique and The Love Meditation. The Witnessing Technique is most beneficial when an individual is in pain, and The Love Meditation is most beneficial when an individual is feeling happy or in love.

The Witnessing Technique

1) Find a strong emotion you want to transform.

2) Allow the emotion to take the form of an image which best represents it.

3) Allow the image to express the emotion in your imagination.

4) Observe what happens without choreographing anything that occurs.

5) Continue to watch the image express itself until the emotion has lost its charge.

6) Once you reach a feeling of neutrality, you will be able to leave the emotion with the image. When this peaceful shift occurs, become aware of the aspect of your consciousness that is able to *observe* the image.

7) Establish your position as the *witness,* by choosing to *identify* with the observant aspect of your consciousness instead of the image.

8) Luxuriate in the empowering feeling of aligning with a higher level of consciousness, instead of remaining trapped in the pain of your programming.

When you are in a negative place, the ego will entice you into *identifying* with your pain. In order to take back control of your power, practice rising above the pain by *dis-identifying* from it. Remember, the pain is only an illusion brought about by the attachments ego has formed. Once you know yourself as the *witness,* (Pure Consciousness) you will never become trapped in the emotional pain of attachment again.

When you apply The Witnessing Technique daily, you will learn to observe the pain with greater clarity. You will understand how it is formed, how to step aside from it, and how to transform it safely. As you establish distance from your negativity, the blissful energy of Pure Consciousness will become more familiar to you than the pain ego projects, and your vibration will accelerate.

The Witnessing Technique is described in greater detail on pages 27-43.

The Love Meditation

To begin The Love Meditation, you must be able to imagine a being for whom you feel unconditional love. A small child you love is often the best choice, but anyone who inspires a powerful feeling of unconditional love will work well. If no one comes to mind, you may choose a pet or imagine an animal that makes you happy, such as a puppy.

When you have the being you love in your awareness, close your eyes and allow yourself to open your heart as much as possible to the love you feel for them. Let your feelings intensify until you have reached a blissful or euphoric state. Sense the energy your love holds and recognize the tremendous expansiveness of its power. Then look within and locate where the *source* of this love is coming from. As you move inside, you will realize that YOU are the source. *In fact, you are the energy itself.*

You will also find that this powerful energy feels stronger and more expansive or real than your physical body. Trust what you are experiencing, and you will rise above the mind's limited view of who and what you are. Once you feel confident with this meditation, you will understand that you have the power of the Universe at your command when you align with your source, which is Pure Love.

Stilling the Mind

You will also have times when you are simply feeling impartial. You may not be riled up enough with negative emotion to apply The Witnessing Technique, and not quite happy enough to apply The Love Mediation. At these times, it is still important to maintain authority over your mind and align with Pure Consciousness.

Most of our energy is consumed by the mind's needless chatter. It runs us around in circles while it focuses on problems, chores, lists, memories, things that bother us, and others that enchant us. Much like a mischievous child, the mind cannot get away with coloring on the walls if we are able to monitor what it is doing. Once you are able to observe the mind without getting caught up in the ideas or emotions it projects, your thoughts will eventually stop and it will become apparent that YOU are the one in control, and the mind need not run your life and dictate your thoughts any longer.

When the mind is still, Pure Consciousness is able to transmit blocks of information that will guide you toward unprecedented success, growth, and happiness in your life. When you receive this information, you can direct the mind according to the insights you are given. The mind must be still, however, in order for the information to come through clearly and be understood.

Historically, this inner guidance has been named "the inner voice," but no words will actually be received. The inner voice is not a voice at all. It is energetic insight and added vitality. Voices or words people hear inside are of the ego and mind. Ego speaks through words: Pure Consciousness communicates through creative energy, which uplifts and delights. This inspiration can later be translated into words and actions, but it arrives first energetically.

If you become frustrated while watching the mind, allow your frustration to form into an image and move into The Witnessing Technique. Each day it will become easier to take control back from your mind and rise above its mundane activities.

The point of this exercise is to know that as the observer of your thoughts and emotions, you are not the mind. Who is the observer if it is not the mind? The observer is Pure Consciousness. Know your greater self as that.

Uplifting Emotional Vibration

Just as electricity flowing through a circuit creates luminous energy to shine through a light bulb, Pure Consciousness flowing through a physical body will infuse a being with positive or light filled emotions, such as openness, self-acceptance, inner peace, playfulness, excitement, unconditional love, and bliss.

When the electric circuit to a light bulb is shut off, the light bulb is dead and dark. When we block the flow of Pure Consciousness, we experience inner darkness of our own in the form of painful emotions, such as shame, guilt, depression, grief, fear, longing, weakness or anger. The ego puts us in a closed position vibrationally.

A negative emotion is simply an indication that your ego is in control or that you are moving toward a lower or destructive vibration. A positive emotion is an indication that Pure Consciousness is flowing freely and you are in alignment with your source. If you are in a negative space, whatever you are doing or whatever is bringing you into that space is igniting the ego. Either move away from that thing, activity or person—or look deeply into what fear this circumstance brings up—so that you can rise above it.

When you feel a positive vibration, open to that feeling more. Vibrational qualities are meant to guide you so that you remain in alignment with Pure Consciousness. If you feel bad, you are out of alignment. If you feel good, you are in harmony with your source.

Daily Meditations for Inner Peace

In cases of trauma or intense shock, moving the eyes rapidly from left to right will lighten up the intensity of the emotion. Rapid eye movement literally uplifts dense energy by massaging the brain, causing a higher frequency of brain activity, raising your mental energy to align more with happiness. This happens naturally during the R.E.M. segments of our sleep, which is why we awaken feeling refreshed.

If you find that your emotions are constantly heavy and you would like to reclaim your energy, an eye movement meditation can be of great benefit. Lay down with your eyes open, making sure that your lips are slightly apart so that the jaws can relax. Move the eyes around in a circle clockwise as fast as possible without straining until you need to stop. Then close your eyes and follow the energy inside. You will find that your focus naturally moves toward the pineal gland in the center of the brain. This gland is the calm space amid the storm of your thoughts and emotions. Bringing your focus to this point regularly will strengthen your connection with Pure Consciousness and contribute a deep sense of inner peace to your life.

Uplifting Mental Vibration

We have a quality to our being that can be described as zeal. You may have noticed people who appear radiant, confident, accomplished, fascinating, and powerful. They seem to exist with some luminous influence. This is zeal. Zeal is a natural part of our inheritance as humans, but we can deplete our zeal easily if the mind takes control of our energy.

When we waste our energy obsessing, judging, or fighting with others, or when we try to impress people in order to receive attention or praise, our zeal becomes depleted.

When our attention is focused outward, we lose energy and vitality.
When our attention is focused inward, we increase our energy and vitality.

As you spend time within—getting to know yourself, appreciating and understanding your internal energy—your vitality will blossom, your intelligence will expand, and you will become radiant with Life Force. Simply bring your mental energy within more often and become interested in the deeper realms of your own energetic world. Once your zeal increases, you will find it easier to maintain a positive outlook on life, even while you are under stress.

Because our source is literally pure bliss, we want to mimic the positive energy of Pure Consciousness in order to align with it vibrationally, which is why we want to train the mind to be as positive as possible when it is active. Using our imagination is often the best way to accomplish this.

When we direct the mind with visions that excite and delight us, we are stimulating very high levels of positive mental energy. Prolonging this sort of rapture will allow the mind to shift into a more creative position and make it easier to maintain an optimistic outlook and to focus on solutions.

When stress does occur, immediately decide that something uplifting will arise from your situation. Next, imagine the most rewarding outcome and instruct your mind to remain focused on that positive vision. You will find that this transforms any negative energy rapidly, and your future events will be more likely to produce a deep sense of fulfillment and happiness.

Uplifting *Physical Vibration*

The totality of your energy is like a torch to unconsciousness. When you bring all your energy into each moment, you become a bright light, and everything becomes clear. People who live deeply reach a level of maturity or transformation that is profoundly different from the masses. They stand apart as original, unique, and authentic—even magical at times.

You must dive into the joy of physical reality with totality in order to bypass the mind. When you bring your total energy into each act, you will know the depths and the heights possible. Walking on the beach, be aware of each step, each breath you take, each sensation you feel. Open to the smell of the ocean, the tingle of the breeze on your skin, the roar of the waves in your ears, the temperature of the sand on your feet. This totality increases your awareness and raises your vibration. We must experience the totality of any moment to really live that moment and know ourselves through it. This "knowing" is a key to our transformation.

The Body

The human body is 80% - 90% water, which is a powerful conductor for the electric current of our Life Force. When we consume fresh, clean water, we offer the best physical conduit to our source.

Like water, oxygen is also a conduit for Pure Consciousness. When we inhale deeply, we allow more Life Force in. When we exhale forcefully, we let out stagnation. This is one reason exercise is so important for our total well being.

The fastest way to diffuse a negative emotion is to exhale forcefully. If you find yourself in trauma, take small breaths in and exhale as forcefully as you can until the extreme energy passes. Then begin to inhale deeply and allow the fresh oxygen to flood your being. You will be surprised how easily you move beyond your pain.

Certain foods lower your vibration, and certain foods raise your vibration. Basically, the more alive, pure, natural, nutrient-rich, easily digestible, water-filled foods hold the highest vibration. The food you eat should also please your palate. Enjoying each meal is a significant ingredient in raising your vibration. Happiness, freedom, and pleasure are very high-vibrational.

Uplifting Environmental Vibration

Nature shows us a quality of life only possible without an ego. In a lush forest, we are surrounded by a world vibrating high above the mind. The neutral energy we find teaches us all we need to know in order to live peacefully and joyously.

A tree will not judge you as good or bad or right or wrong. A flower doesn't care if you are Christian, Muslim, Jewish, black, white, male or female, fat, skinny, rich or poor. Without an ego, no need to judge or impress exists, which is why nature is so alluring and comforting. Nature's beauty stands strong as a constant reminder of our very own source.

Spend time in nature and bring that peaceful quality back with you into your personal space. Even a picture of nature by your desk will stimulate higher vibrations. Looking at a waterfall, an ocean, or a thriving forest can catapult you into a profound state of serenity.

Purification

The elements of nature are constantly purifying and regenerating our planet. To align with this force, we want to mimic its virtues and continually purify our own personal environment as well. Clean, bright, sparkling things have a much higher vibration than dull, gloomy, dirty things. More energy exists in a clean space, because it can flow more easily. The same is true of the body. When it is clean, your Life Force can flow more easily.

To increase the vibration of your environment, it is helpful to clean those areas that accumulate dirt and stagnant energy regularly. Clearing out clutter and cleansing will cause a space to feel more alive and revitalized immediately. Fresh, flowing air is a wonderful energizer as well.

Many ways are open to you to raise the totality of your vibration. Only a few highlights have been covered here. Use your imagination and make it a fun game to come up with more ideas to raise your own vibration with things that make you happy. Design it specifically for yourself, so that every day you will be sure to raise your vibration spiritually, emotionally, mentally, physically, and environmentally, by adding more joy, love, purity, and playfulness to *everything* you do.

Playfulness

Have you ever wondered what makes a person laugh? The unexpected is the reason. We laugh every time the mind is unable to foresee the outcome according to its divisions, certainties, rationale and expectations. The moment the mind is surprised or caught off guard, it stops, and a glimpse of Pure Consciousness can slip in. A laugh is the result. Pure Consciousness is very jolly.

Even when others are angry, cruel, or dramatic, if we can watch them and imagine they are cartoon characters, they will instantly become much less intimidating or offensive. Reflecting on your own ego-driven behavior (by witnessing your symbolic images) will help you take your own mental programming less seriously as well.

More lightheartedness throughout the day keeps the programming disengaged. The longer periods of time you can go without the mind being solemn or serious, the easier it will be to raise your vibration and expand your consciousness. Ego is serious. Pure Consciousness is playful.

Summary

Techniques abound to deprogram, reprogram, modify, alter, revise, hypnotize, psychoanalyze, and adjust the mind. These methods, however, keep the individual focused *in* the mind. To overcome patterning and inappropriate thoughts, beliefs, and behaviors of any sort, we must *rise above* the mind and all its programming. We can easily accomplished this once we connect with the neutral energy of Pure Consciousness by applying The Witnessing Technique, The Love Meditation, stilling the mind, or by living each breath with totality.

Not much is required to manifest in physical reality, but to be a person of great magnificence you must rise above the ego and take back control of your life. Those who flow with uncommon grace and inner beauty and those who inspire us with the radiance of their presence or delight us with unparalleled creativity, are the people who have aligned with their source and discovered the unique magic of their soul.

The following chapters outline real examples of people who have applied these techniques to overcome the mental programming which caused them the most pain. The names and intimate details have been changed to protect their identities.

PART TWO

Case studies of people who applied
The Witnessing Technique
to rise above their painful programming

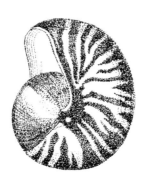

CHAPTER 6

Addiction

Introduction

*Psychological reliance on some outside dependency
that leads an individual to abandon the self.*

R ARELY IS A HUMAN TAUGHT HOW TO DEAL with their most intense fears and emotional traumas, although this is the most important and necessary tool for well-being. When fear and pain arise, our programmed information can at best guide us to move toward something that will momentarily take away our pain, or at least make us forget about it for a while. Drugs, alcohol, and other intoxicants are needed by those who believe they have nowhere else to turn to sooth their aching soul.

Will-power and discipline are no matches for the emptiness our addictions hope to satisfy. We must fill that void with energy that is eternally satisfying. Consequently, the addictive programming will disappear on its own.

The Witnessing Technique offers a tremendous support system *before*, *during*, and *after* abstinence. This technique is specifically intended to triumph over any programming which tethers the addict to their self-destructive patterns. Strong physical and emotion support systems are important compliments to the technique when chemicals are involved.

Chemicals and Higher Consciousness

Many intoxicants are desired for their ability to create a chemically-induced glimpse of higher consciousness. Drugs, such as LSD, Heroine, Ecstasy, Angel Dust, and Cocaine, can occasionally bring the user into a higher reality above the limitations of the mind, by killing the ego. Their experience will feel freeing, expansive, and unlimited, because it creates a glimpse beyond what the mind would normally allow.

Many problems occur, however, when the intoxicants wear off and the users are brought back into the experience of the mind, where they find the familiarity of their ego (old identity) has been shattered. This is similar to a tiny baby waking up as an adult one day and by nightfall, it is back in its "baby reality," carrying with it the experience of having already been an adult. Returning to the mind's previous reality will now feel confusing, limited, and often unbearable.

Although we want to rise above the programming in the mind (ego), to rise above it all at once by shattering the ego is too much of a shock for our system. The ego gives us a bearing on life. It is a false bearing, but nonetheless, we rely on it for our mental stability. We need to rise above this mental structure consciously and at our own pace in order to maintain our sanity.

The Witnessing Technique guides us into a reality beyond the ego in safe but profound increments. Concurrently, we are able to maintain our awareness of the programming (ego.) We can see both realities clearly, and we are able to make a conscious choice concerning which reality we want to *identify* with. Most importantly, we can choose either reality at any time. If we want to allow the programming, we can. If we choose to connect with Pure Consciousness and rise above the programming, we can. With neither threat nor trauma, we have an empowering experience, because we know we are always in control.

Those who reach a glimpse of higher consciousness through drugs are *not* in control. They have neither steering wheel nor brakes, nor do they know how to reach higher levels of consciousness without the use of drugs. Once they fall back into the mind, their lives may turn chaotic as their psyche reaches frantically to recreate a new ego structure that feels real. This is similar to the baby trying to forget they had a glimpse of being an adult. The baby will dive into all the old infant experiences, yet nothing will feel right anymore, so an attempt to construct a new identity; that will be even more fragile than the first one, begins.

After scrambling to reconnect some boundaries and categories with which to live, if the user once again takes the drug, his new identity (ego) will be shattered even more ruthlessly. Pieces of the old ego and fragments of the new structure will be blown apart in the mind, causing further disorientation when the drug wears off. Soon the user will have a totally different personality, or he will lose his bearing on reality altogether. A schizophrenic mind begins to occur. A mind unable to grasp which reality it is in.

It is impossible to reach Enlightenment or maintainable levels of higher consciousness through the use of drugs. Hallucinogens may appear to be a short cut, however, they actually retard the healthy expansion of consciousness by leaving the user with a much stronger attachment to his ego as the mind scrambles to give him some sense of stability. Unfortunately, the user may not even be aware that drugs have altered his mental capacity or level of awareness. He will grasp onto the mind, desperately clinging to what he sees as his reality, often assuming that everyone else is crazy and he is sane. A grandiose or antisocial personality may form

A more comprehensive glimpse of higher consciousness (than the one reached through drugs) can be easily reached through regular practice of The Witnessing Technique or The Love Meditation. There is no need to experiment with drugs in an attempt to reach a euphoric level of consciousness. It is within us already.

A Note to the Seasoned Drug User

If you have used drugs extensively, this information is important for you. When you practice The Witnessing Technique, remain connected to the aspect of your consciousness that is able to watch the images your emotions form in your mind. If you have drug flash backs or hallucinations, do the same thing. *Remain identified with the aspect of your consciousness that is able to witness what you see or feel while you are hallucinating.* Do this to the best of your ability, even if it sounds impossible. As you practice, life will begin to feel more within your control as you learn to anchor your consciousness in one dimension.

Witnessing: A Path to Overcome Addiction to Alcohol

Henry was a great athlete, but he failed to make the final cut for pro football. When he received the news, he went on a drinking binge in New Orleans and did not stop until he passed out two days later. When Henry regained consciousness, he discovered that he was married to his high school sweetheart, a girl he had brought along for the fun. His new wife became pregnant while they were there, so Henry decided to find an alternate way to earn a good living. He received his real estate license within six months and began selling properties right away. The hours were demanding, however, so he kept himself going with a little cocaine and a lot of martinis.

On Henry's twenty-third birthday, he decided to celebrate in Las Vegas with a few of his buddies, and left his wife alone with the baby. Two months after Henry's birthday trip, he received a portfolio of pictures that proved he had been sexually active with a showgirl on his first night in town, along with a note claiming that she was pregnant. Henry went straight to a bar, and when he stumbled into his house at 4:00 a.m., he left his briefcase outside of the entry way. When his wife picked it up to bring it inside, the briefcase fell open, and all the Las Vegas pictures spilled out onto the floor. Knowing that this was not the first time Henry had experimented with extramarital sex, his wife left him the next day, taking their child with her.

Abandoning all his responsibilities, Henry immediately embarked upon a six day binge. On the seventh day he showed up at his office, only to be served with divorce papers. Henry launched right into another binge, which ended when he woke up in the hospital with two broken legs after wrapping his Porsche around a tree. Most of the friends who came to visit him in the hospital were pro football players or very successful businessmen with happy families. Henry was glad to see them, but the visits created a painful contrast in relation to his own life.

When he was released from the hospital, a real-estate colleague suggested The Witnessing Technique, so Henry made an appointment. He arrived for his first session with the smell of alcohol on his breath and sweat pouring off his large face. Henry shared what had happened in his life and how ready he was to "remain focused," as he put it. When it came time to access his emotions, however, he felt numb to his present life conditions. He was unwilling to talk about his divorce, so he was guided to recreate the emotions he felt the day he learned that he had not made the cut for pro football. Henry instantly bowed his head and covered his eyes with his huge hands, sharing that he felt like a complete failure. He had partied too hard the last week of recruits, which hindered his performance. He was still upset for having let himself down.

Henry was guided to allow the feelings he had to form into an image in his mind, and the vision of a three-year-old boy standing in front of a very tall, heavy door appeared. Henry watched the child as he tried to open the door, but the handle was too high.

Henry chuckled and commented that it reminded him of the last time he had ever seen his father. With his eyes still closed, Henry recalled a vicious fight his mother and father had over his father's infidelity when Henry was only three-years-old. Henry recalled running into the room just as his father was rushing out and being hit in the head with the opening door. His father did not stop to see if he was all right. Instead, he slammed the door behind him, never to return. Henry tried to get the door open to run after his father, but he couldn't. The handle was too high, and his mother would not help. His father was killed in a car accident a few months later, so he never saw him again.

Henry was quiet for a long while and then he chuckled again and said, "I have not thought about that since the day it happened." Then he shared that the door seemed like *The End* and that the little boy was not clever enough or tall enough to get through. *He was not enough,* and it had cost him. There was nothing he could do about it.

Even though the boy in Henry's mind was a vision of himself as a child, the image was still viewed symbolically in order to access how his mind perceived the incident. Henry was then guided to close his eyes and allow the image to express his pain for him. The boy bowed his head and began to cry, because he did not think he was important enough for anyone to care about him. *Henry's mind had become convinced that he was not enough the day his father left.* He also felt there must be something wrong with him to be left behind. Whenever he was sad about his father being gone, his mother would often scream, "What is wrong with you?" which engrained the programming even further.

Henry agreed to watch the image on his own during the week, and when he arrived for his next session, he shared that he had thought a lot about not believing he measured up, only to conclude that all the success he had achieved in his life was due to this idea. He felt it made him strive for more. Because of this, he was very resistant to rising above his programming.

Henry was guided to close his eyes and allow the feeling of not being enough to form into an image, and once again the vision of a three-year-old boy appeared. He allowed the image to express his fear of *not being enough* until the emotion had lost its charge, then he was guided to connect with the aspect of his consciousness that was able to observe the image of the boy. Once Henry had identified with his *Witnessing Self,* his entire body positioning shifted, and he grew a wide smile. He shared that from this new perspective, he could see that the boy was more than enough; even if the image itself would always believe otherwise. Henry also realized that his *Witnessing Self* was actually his *authentic self* before the programming had entered his mind. From the fresh perspective of his *Witnessing Self,* Henry felt invincible. Without his core fear of not being enough, he knew he could accomplish anything and maintain his success.

Henry spent some time elaborating on how powerful he felt once he was able to detach from his programming. Then he was asked if his *Witnessing Self* felt the need to drink or take drugs in order to escape the pain, and he answered no. As the *witness,* he was merely an observer; removed from the pain, and he had no need to escape through drinking or drugs. His fear of not being enough was the only driving force behind his desire for alcohol.

Henry had stopped using cocaine after his accident, but he was still drinking heavily. Brief periods of abstinence from liquor had caused him to feel empty and lost, which created an even greater desire for alcohol, as well as a hopeless feeling that he would always be dependent on it. Now that Henry had been introduced to his *Witnessing Self,* he felt capable of overcoming any dependency.

When Henry was ready to face his alcoholism, he was not asked to cut back on his alcohol intake. Instead, he was given the option of continuing to drink as much as he wanted, but to become extremely aware every time he saw himself moving toward his dependency. All he had to do was watch what emotion or impulse motivated him to drink.

Henry practiced this technique for one week and returned frustrated, sharing that whenever he wanted a drink, he became extremely uncomfortable when he tuned into his motivating emotions. He discovered that he could not be aware and take a drink at the same time, so he had given up on being aware, and continued to drink unconsciously. Something inside of Henry had already shifted, however, and he was unable to drink to the point of passing out. He would stop after a few drinks and then get busy doing something else.

There is a powerful force that is always at work uplifting us, carrying us to higher ground, if only we open to it. The Witnessing Technique creates this opening. Once Henry agreed to be more aware, he opened the door to higher levels of consciousness that could assist him. He was no longer alone with his pain and addiction.

Henry also shared that his new found emotions were causing him to feel nervous and frazzled. In the past he would have drowned his irritation in a martini, but a growing "inner sense" told him that more alcohol would only contribute additional stress to his life. To escape his uneasiness, Henry spent more time with his physical therapist strengthening his legs. That seemed to help a bit, but he was still overwhelmed with anxiety.

Most addicts experience a difficult transitional period when the program-ming tries to fight to maintain control. If this happens, clients are guided to continue practicing the technique without judging themselves. They may experi-ence an uncomfortable stage where nothing feels quite right, but soon they will reach a connection to their Witnessing Self which lifts them above the pain and confusion. If they keep moving forward, Pure Consciousness will carry them the rest of the way.

Henry was congratulated on his progress, and then he was guided to allow the anxious energy he felt to form into an image in his mind. When he closed his eyes, the vision of a video game ball zipping all over the place appeared. The video game ball had no direction or destination. It simply zipped around until it hit a barrier, and then it changed course and zipped into the next wall. Henry watched the ball and expressed that it was looking for a way out, but there was no escaping the chaos.

Henry allowed the ball to zip around until he felt neutral about the anxiety the ball represented. Then he was guided to connect with the aspect of his consciousness that was able to observe the ball. Once Henry had identified with his *Witnessing Self*, he was able to recognize that the ball represented a program in his mind which caused him to believe there was no way out of his pain. His programming convinced him to go full force ahead in any direction until he was knocked down.

From the Witnessing position, Henry could see that his mind had no solution for his anxiety; it only exhausted and frustrated him further. As the *witness*, however, Henry experienced no anxiety at all. He felt removed from the image and the pain. He realized that he had the choice to iden-tify with the calm, observant aspect of himself, his *Witnessing Self*, or he could zip around and hit his head against every wall he encountered. Henry agreed to watch this image every time he felt anxious, then identify with the aspect of his consciousness that was able to *observe* the anxiety, instead of becoming it.

On his ninth session Henry came in looking upset, sharing that his ex-wife had announced that she was planning to marry someone else within a few months. Henry was attached to the idea that they would get back together as a family, so her news devastated him. The first thing he wanted to do was drink, but he had not done that yet. Something inside of him felt sick at the thought of moving into a pattern that had caused his pain in the first place. He was beginning to wake up to the truth and face it with awareness instead of relying on his old patterns.

Henry was guided to close his eyes and allow the pain he felt to form into an image, and the vision of a small boy standing in front of a closed door once again appeared. The child felt that anyone who ever meant anything to him would always choose to walk out of the door and never look back, because he was not important enough for them to want to stay. He was just not enough.

Once he was able to identify with his *Witnessing Self*, Henry recognized that he could give into the programming and live his life according to this fear, or he could rise above the programming and watch it, without allowing it to control his idea of how his life would play out.

With newfound confidence, Henry decided to face the emotions his ex-wife brought up for him each time they arose, no matter how painful that might be. Rising above the pain of this programming (not being enough) was a turning point in his life, because it was the pivotal idea around which his addictive personality revolved. *When we face our most rigid programming, it can never have the same intense control over us again.*

After a few days of practicing the technique, Henry was surprised to realize that he was capable of making the choice to *witness* his program-ming, instead of allowing it to run his life. He was willing to rise above the belief that he would always be left alone and in pain because he was not enough. *Once we are able to see the programming clearly, it begins to look absurd. It is only when it is hidden in our subconscious that it can determine our destiny.*

When Henry arrived for his next appointment, he expressed that he had no desire to drink after watching his images all week. This had come as quite a shock to him since he had been so close to bingeing the week before. Now, every time he thought of alcohol, his stomach turned sour, and he would become uncomfortable. When this occurred, he would *witness* his anxious video game ball image, and rise above the programming instead of being controlled by it. To his surprise, it worked, and his anxiety disappeared each time.

Choosing to *witness* his pain, instead of escape it, was not the easiest choice for Henry to make, but something authentic had been awakened inside which supported him in moving forward with this new behavior. *It is important to understand that Henry did not suppress his urge to drink. Another part of his consciousness, which had no interest in alcohol, was starting to take over. He was being supported by an **awakened** energy deep within.*

When Henry arrived for his next appointment, he was quite happy with his progress, but he had some concern that eventually he would fall back into his unconscious habit of reaching for a drink every time stressful emotions arose. Henry was guided to allow this new fear to form into an image, and a weakling nerd appeared. The nerd was afraid of life, because everything appeared more powerful than he was. He had no control over anything around him. Henry watched the programming and realized that he could choose to allow the image to run his life and make him believe that he had no power to deal with anything, or he could *dis-identify* from the weakling and *witness* the image, *instead of becoming him.*

Henry chuckled, sharing that he had no intention of allowing a weakling kid to control his life and make him drink. He left the session feeling self-assured, and when he returned one month later, he reported that he had neither taken a drink nor had he wanted to. Henry laughed and said, "Once I saw that weakling kid, not even the best booze in the world could get me excited. I don't want to be some weakling."

Henry made amends with his ex-wife, and she agreed to give him visiting rights with his child. He has confidence that his relationship with his son will grow and last, unlike his relationship with his own father. Henry has been sober for over twelve years as of this publishing. More importantly, staying sober has not been a struggle for him. He has a higher level of consciousness that helps him feel good enough just as he is and powerful enough to face any pain as the *witness*.

Witnessing: A Path to Overcome
Addiction to Prescription Drugs

Jason's IQ was so high that many of the professors at his Ivy League University wanted to meet him. After receiving his Masters degree, he became involved with space travel and higher technology. He had three major relationships in his life, and when the last one ended, he decided never to venture into areas of the heart again. He felt much more comfortable in his head where he knew he did well.

Spending a significant amount of time alone, however, caused Jason's mind to become extremely overactive. His constant analyzing of numbers and ideas made it almost impossible for him to sleep. After months of insomnia, his health and energy began to suffer, so his physician put him on a mild sedative, which helped him sleep for about one week. Not only was he able to sleep, but the constant headache which followed him around was also gone. By the second week of using his prescription, however, Jason started feeling *fuzzy* and he was unable to remain focused at work. The side effect infuriated him, because he took pride in having a clear mind that could calculate solutions at lightning speed.

Jason went back to his doctor to ask for a prescription that was less potent, but instead his doctor gave him another prescription for mental clarity and alertness. Jason took the sleeping pill at night and the "alert" pills in the morning and found that he was more awake and clear. Within one month, however, Jason developed a nervous tick around his left eye which made him appear a bit like a mad scientist. This frustrated him while he was working and embarrassed him around his co-workers. Jason went back to his doctor with concern that his nervous tick was caused by a reaction to one of the drugs he had been taking, but his doctor insisted on giving him yet another prescription that would affect his nervous system and calm his reflexes down.

Jason took all three medications for three months, but the nervous tick did not go away, so he discontinued using all the drugs. Within one week his nervous tick had disappeared, but once again he was unable to sleep. A co-worker offered him something that he had been taking to help him sleep. Jason tried the new drug, and it worked well—no nervous ticks and no grogginess in the morning. The new drug, however, made Jason much more irritable. Another colleague offered him a drug that would make him "happy," so he tried it that night and found that he was very mellow when he took the drug and also more interested in finding a female partner.

Jason went out that evening to a bar and met a woman who took him back to her place. He started a relationship with her and continued to take more of the "happy drug," in order to sedate his fear of intimacy. He also received additional prescriptions to enhance his sexual performance, help him relax, and keep him alert. Jason added more chemicals as the year continued, until he was taking up to eight different drugs a day, just to keep his body functioning the way he wanted it to. After six months, however, most of the helpful effects of these drugs had worn off, and Jason was left despondent. His doctor subsequently put him on antidepressants to counteract his lack of verve.

During the holiday season, Jason injured himself on the job. Once the emergency care unit had received a list of all the drugs Jason had in his system, he was sent to a facility that could help him detoxify from the incompatible chemicals. After his release, Jason was clear-minded and healthy, but he felt insecure about his ability to deal with life without the use of the prescriptions on which he had previously depended. Jason's sister suggested he begin working with The Witnessing Technique, adding that it might help him relax without the use of drugs. That sounded exciting, so he made an appointment.

When Jason arrived for his session, he shared that the emotion with which he had the most difficulty, was the feeling of powerlessness. When he was guided to close his eyes and allow his feelings to form into an image, the vision of a meek boy sitting in a corner wearing a dunce hat appeared. Jason described the boy as timid and frightened. The only power he trusted was his own intelligence, but even that seemed to be in jeopardy sitting in the corner with a dunce cap on. Jason commented that if the boy was not able to prove to others that he was valuable and useful in a very unique way, that no one would respect him. In order to avoid being controlled, overpowered, or used, the boy's only hope was to silently outsmart everyone.

Jason compared what he found in the image with his daily life and admitted that in order to feel good about himself, he needed to display a unique value at work and never make a mistake. According to his programming, he had to maintain his genius status at all times, or he would end up like the boy in his image, powerless and humiliated. Once Jason felt neutral about the image, he was guided to connect with the aspect of his consciousness that was able to observe the character. He identified with his *Witnessing Self* quite easily and instantly felt free from the insecurities and fears that the boy in his image represented. This new perspective on life infused Jason with a tremendous sense of inner peace and self-confidence.

When Jason arrived for his next appointment, he shared that he had experienced difficulty sleeping the night after his first session, so he applied The Witnessing Technique on his own. The emotion he felt while tossing and turning was frustration, so he closed his eyes and allowed his frustration to form into an image, and once again the boy with the dunce hat appeared. Jason soon realized that he was acting just like the boy in his image, feeling insecure about his status at work, desperate to prove he was valuable. Once Jason recognized the programming, he was able to *witness* the image of the boy and detach from it. Instantly, the turmoil of the character no longer had any relation to him, so he was able to relax and let go. He was neither the boy, nor was he useless or helpless. He was the *witness*. This worked wonderfully for Jason, and he was finally able to get to sleep without the use of sleeping pills.

On his third session, Jason wanted to investigate the programming which caused his aversion to relationships. Intimacy brought up fear that he would eventually be rejected no matter how valuable or useful he proved he could be to a partner. Jason closed his eyes and allowed his fear to form into an image, and the vision of a lone puzzle piece that did not fit with the rest of the puzzle arose. Jason felt that he was too different to be accepted or loved. When he disconnected from the image, (by identifying with his *Witnessing Self*), he felt a sudden shift occur. Without the programming standing in the way of his true essence, he was able to enjoy his individuality and feel an authentic appreciation for the way he was.

As Jason continued to practice The Witnessing Technique, he became much more confident in general. He began a new relationship with a woman who was very loving, and he never felt the need to use prescription drugs to enhance his sexual performance or to relax around her. Once Jason had risen above his core fear, he felt comfortable in all situations. By utilizing the power within, he no longer had any need for drugs.

Witnessing: A Path to Overcome

Addiction to Hallucinogenic Drugs

Sandra never understood why her family saw her as a delinquent. She did well in school, she was a member of the band and drama club, and she had a lot of friends. Sandra's parents, however, did not like the fact that she enjoyed dyeing her hair a different color each month. She also had some tattoos and piercings; all signs to her parents that she was a lost cause. They felt embarrassed by her and condemned her for her different choices every chance they had.

Sandra ran away from home at a young age, certain this would make her feel better about herself, because she saw her family as the root of her pain. Desperately wanting to find a support system of people who would accept her, Sandra passed through many towns reaching out to others with her story. One night she met an older man named Nick who invited her over to his apartment. He offered her a joint of marijuana, so she took a puff and gave it back. Although Sandra had consciously stayed away from drugs in the past, at this point in her life, she found the drug comforting. Once she relaxed, her problems began to feel far away. Nick offered her a warm place to stay for as long as she needed, and Sandra felt she had finally met someone who accepted and understood her.

As time went on, Nick began asking her for favors, such as delivering bags of marijuana to buyers and picking up packages from warehouses. It was not long before he introduced her to cocaine, which eventually gave him more power over her than she felt comfortable giving him. Her emotions became more tumultuous each day, as her self-hatred continued to rise. She contemplated suicide, and many times she would cut herself as self-punishment, leaving scars all over her arms and legs. In another attempt to feel free, she pierced her nose, shaved her head, and started wearing nothing but black, affirming her independence from society.

One evening Sandra was strung out wandering the streets, when she stepped in front of an oncoming car and landed in the hospital with a broken hip. She woke up in a room beside a very pleasant older woman who began telling Sandra all about her life. The woman mentioned how much she had loved her daughter, but that her daughter had died when she was only seventeen. Sandra felt close to someone for the first time in years. She wanted to take the place of her daughter and finally have someone who would love her in her life.

Once Sandra was released from the hospital, she was placed in a half way house for homeless teens grappling with drug addiction. She was given a strong support system that helped her with her physical cravings for drugs, and she met quite a few new friends there. She also found a job as a ticket taker and started saving her money. After one month of sobriety, Sandra's friend from the hospital told her about The Witnessing Technique and offered to pay for her sessions, so she agreed.

When Sandra arrived for her appointment, she began to cry while she expressed how much she had always hated herself, commenting that her only purpose in life was to be the scapegoat for everyone else's unhealed pain. Other people's opinions of her had affected her so deeply that she had become someone very different from who she had intended to be.

Sandra recalled a time in her childhood when she had been out of town with her school band for the weekend when a diamond ring went missing from a neighbor's house. Everyone's first reaction was that Sandra had taken it. The ring was eventually found, because it had only been misplaced by the owner, but no one in her family apologized for their accusations. Sandra could not imagine how they ever began to view her as a delinquent in the first place.

Sandra closed her eyes and allowed the feeling of being bad to form into an image in her mind, and the vision of a black sheep appeared. The sheep was weak and shy, and it stood in the background. The other sheep were white and free. The black sheep had been condemned by the whole herd, and there was no denying it was different, because it was black and the others were white.

According to Sandra's programming, everything that made her original and unique also made her unacceptable and disconnected. This realization brought up anger, which formed into the vision of a crazy looking Ninja. The Ninja had a knife poised ready to attack himself on command. He beat his chest until it was bloody, stabbed at his thighs, threw himself up against the wall, pulled out his hair, and punched his body all over until he passed out. *This image represented how Sandra used self-punishment to vent her anger.*

Sandra continued to watch the image and allowed her emotions to disperse through the Ninja's violent attacks. Soon the anger appeared to be something the image was experiencing, but it no longer felt attached to her. She was then guided to connect with the aspect of her consciousness that was able to observe the image, and once she had identified with her *Witnessing Self,* she expressed relief at being able to detach from her inner rage and embrace herself the way she was.

When Sandra returned for her next session, she shared that she had been observing her images all week, and she had come to the conclusion that the Ninja was only following orders from some outside authority. He expected to be rewarded, even if it meant he had to kill himself first. He just wanted to please the authority. *Sandra believed that her parents (the authority figures in her life) wanted her to feel badly about herself, and the only way to appease them was to do so. The more she destroyed herself, the more she hoped she would be pleasing her parents. If she pleased them, she hoped they would make her feel safe and secure one day.* Sandra also recognized that no one expected her to do well. She believed that if she did well, she would be in even worse standing with her family. She had to play the role of the delinquent in order to keep everyone happy about the people *they* were.

When the full extent of these realizations appeared in Sandra's awareness, she immediately wanted to get high. She then realized that was exactly what the programming forced her to do, so that she would continue to appear bad and inferior to the rest of her family. This infuriated her so much that she flushed her (hidden reserve) pot down the toilet. Then she spent all her saved-up, cocaine money on a new outfit and a good meal for herself and came home feeling a victory had occurred. For once she had not punished herself under the influence of stressful emotions. From that point forward, Sandra no longer had the desire to turn to drugs when she felt upset or angry.

When Sandra did feel self-destructive energy arising, she would observe the image of the Ninja and allow the character to act out the self-destructive behavior, instead of physically harming herself. In order to anchor her new self-loving response to life, she would move toward a positive, self-nurturing act; such as going for a walk or taking a bath at the end of the day. She was breaking the old programming by remaining the *witness* of it and behaving differently. As Sandra continued to apply The Witnessing Technique to rise above her patterns, she eventually felt a sense of compassion for her family.

Once Sandra had reached a strong level of self-acceptance, she stopped cutting herself with knives when she was upset, and she no longer felt attracted to any chemical support. Instead, she wanted to create something wonderful for herself. Her old programming had convinced her that she would always be a failure, but from the *witnessing perspective*, life appeared to be an opportunity for adventure and success.

As time went on, Sandra's appearance changed drastically. She let her hair grow, she began wearing bright, happy colors, and a beautiful smile appeared on her face. For the first time in many years, Sandra felt good about herself. She worked so diligently with The Witnessing Technique, that she no longer experiences pain regarding her childhood, and she has been drug free for eighteen years, as of this publishing.

Witnessing: A Path to Overcome
Addiction to Smoking

After smoking his first cigarette at the age of ten, Clive found that he was restless and on edge without the smoke of a cigarette swirling around him. By the time he had graduated from college, he was up to eight packages of cigarettes a day. His habit was of no concern to him until he turned thirty and met Mary, the girl of his dreams. Mary did not smoke, and the only thing holding her back from agreeing to marry Clive was his chain smoking.

During the first few months of dating Mary, Clive had no difficulty cutting back to four packages a day without trying. For this reason, he did not think quitting altogether would be difficult. *Since all our programming is in the mind, it is common for our addictions to lose some control over us when we move into the heart, as in the case of opening to love.* Determined to quit altogether, Clive engaged the use of many advertised products, which seemed to help him suppress his desire for a cigarette for one or two weeks at a time. During these periods, however, he became extremely childish and dependent on Mary, which put a strain on their relationship.

Nine times over a two-year period, Clive quit smoking and then started again. The added stress and self-criticism caused him to reach for other soothing vices, such as beer, junk food, and television. Due to these added comforts, Clive put on sixty-three pounds.

Mary was very compassionate and active in searching for a method that would help Clive quit smoking. When she discovered The Witnessing Technique, she introduced it to Clive, and they both felt it would be helpful for their relationship, as well as Clive's addiction.

Since Mary was also working with the technique, she agreed to be supportive of Clive in every way she could, which meant no punishing comments, no pointing out when she saw him smoking, no complaining about his smoky smell, and no pressure about his progress. Her support was a great help to Clive, because he did not have the added pressure of someone else's expectations, which could have led to more self-condemnation. Clive agreed to refrain from his criticism of Mary as well. Not only did their mutual respect help raise their level of awareness, but their relationship improved dramatically.

When Clive spoke, his voice was very labored. He sounded much like Darth Vader in between sentences. When he opened up about his addiction, Clive expressed that smoking had been a good friend and a great comfort to him. In fact, whenever he was without a cigarette, he experienced a sense of abandonment and panic. He also expressed there was something about his labored breathing that felt soothing. He joked that it reminded him that he was still alive.

Clive was guided to close his eyes and allow the intensity of his panic to form into an image, and the vision of a tiny baby in an incubator appeared. The thick oxygen in the tank was misty and white, and the child was gasping for air. In Clive's mind, the baby had a meek broken cry that sounded frightening and desperate. As he continued to watch the image, he suddenly remembered spending three weeks in an incubator himself. He had never thought much about his difficult birth or the perilous weeks he hung on for life, but now he found he was reliving his childhood experience with intense clarity.

As he watched the image of the child in the tank, Clive sensed that no one had come to touch, cuddle, or love him. The closest thing to comfort was the thickness of the air that surrounded him, as well as the labored sound of the oxygen pumping through his tank. The thick swirling air was what he recognized as love and safety. *Smoking cigarettes was the closest he could come to re-enacting his first sense of safety when he lingered on the verge of death for three weeks in the incubator.*

As Clive continued to watch the image of the baby gasping for air, he noticed that it was not air it really wanted. It yearned for touch and love. Clive thought back to the sporadic few weeks he had gone without a cigarette and how needy he had become for constant attention, touch, and love from his girlfriend. He did not want to let her out of his sight, which made her feel smothered. Without his cigarettes, he simply became dependent on Mary instead.

Clive spent the next two weeks observing the tiny baby in the incubator in his mind. Every time he practiced *witnessing*, his identification with the baby and its pain and neediness diminished. As his attachment decreased, his desire to smoke decreased as well.

During this time, Clive discovered that he was not attached to smoking itself, he was attached to swirling smoke and the sound of labored breathing. His most comforting feeling in the past had been sitting in his big delivery truck with the windows rolled up, until he filled his whole vehicle with thick gray swirling smoke. The dense blanket of smoke felt "better than sex" in Clive's words.

On his fifth session, Clive was determined to overcome his attachment to the sound of labored breathing and swirling thick smoke. The feeling that surfaced when he imagined being deprived of his smoky experience, was discomfort. Clive closed his eyes and allowed the feeling of discomfort to form into an image, and the vision of the baby in the incubator appeared again. Once Clive had reached a neutral feeling about the baby, he was guided to identify with his *Witnessing Self* and share the difference he experienced within these two perspectives, (the witness and the ego.) As the *witness*, Clive experienced a new sense of power; his Life Force felt eternal and infinite. When he identified with his ego-programming, he experienced terror that life could be extinguished at any moment.

Clive was then asked if his witnessing experience felt powerful enough to replace the programmed comfort on which he was dependent (the thick air and labored breathing), and he was surprised to find that his experience of safety and comfort were much more significant as the *witness*.

As Clive continued to practice The Witnessing Technique, he was able to identify with the peaceful energy of his *Witnessing Self* more consistently, and he could anchor the comfort he found. Very soon, Clive was able to put down his pack of cigarettes almost every time he reached for them. Only at night when he was very tired and unaware and when his stress level was a bit higher, he chose **not** to use The Witnessing Technique and opted for a cigarette instead.

After a few weeks, however, something very interesting happened. While Clive was smoking his evening cigarette, it tasted terrible. He found himself choking on the smoke and putting the cigarette out before he had finished it. He was grumpy for a few days, because he realized that he could no longer find the illusion of comfort in a cigarette. *That pattern had been weakened, so the programming was no longer able to fool his senses.* The true experience that his body had while he smoked a cigarette had been revealed to him.

Clive continued to *try* to smoke to get the old feeling back. Eventually he gave up and began moving toward his *Witnessing Self* as his sole source of comfort. He was anxious and angry through this transition and his mind put up a tough fight. However, Clive's connection to the truth pulled him over the top, and his mind could only annoy him. It could no longer seduce him into his old behavior.

When you become angry or frustrated during a detox, this is the most impor-tant time to be self supportive. The mind is a poor loser. In order to avoid its tantrums, do something fun as you ride it out. The more you identify with Pure Consciousness, the less the mind can come in to disturb your progress.

After only a few months, Clive no longer had *any* craving to smoke, but he still felt a bit odd without holding a cigarette in his hand. He was encouraged to do something playful with a cigarette in order to break the physical habit of wanting to hold onto them. He chose to pretend he was a magician who could make the cigarettes disappear while Mary joyfully watched his shows. Soon, the serious habit of needing to have a cigarette in his hand for comfort was replaced by the joy of being playful and using it for magic tricks. After three days of his playful routine, Clive never felt the need to hold or have a cigarette again.

Clive and Mary embarked upon an exercise routine and took long hikes and bike rides in the hills. Clive's lungs healed quickly, and he was able to breath freely within six months. Excited by his new found energy, he decided to train for a marathon. Mary and Clive ran together after eleven months of training, and they both finished the race.

Once Clive committed to The Witnessing Technique, he not only released his addictive need for cigarette smoking, he also lost 72 pounds. Clive now has the ability to find love, safety, and comfort within himself, instead of being dependent on an outside source. His connection to Pure Consciousness provided a new identity and a new way of life.

Witnessing: A Path to Overcome
Sexual Addiction

Rick was a musician in a rock and roll band. He traveled all over the world and had no problem finding multiple partners in each new city. After touring on and off for five years, Rick estimated that he had engaged in sex with over five thousand people. Sometimes he would sleep with five or six people at once or have sex with three or four different people in one day.

Everything about life was sexual to Rick. He enjoyed using words in a sexual manner, and he was able to turn any topic of conversation into a sexual dialogue. His jokes, gestures, and even his answering machine message and Christmas cards were blatantly sexual in nature. Although Rick was forty-one years old, he still dressed and acted as if he were a teenager. He chose his hairstyle, car, house, and furnishings with the intent to encourage sexual encounters. The only reason to be alive, in Rick's mind, was to have great sex.

One day after a very exhausting tour, Rick noticed a bloody looking bruise on his neck. He thought it had to be a hickey from some of the groupies he had slept with the night before, but instead of going away while he took time off to rest, another one appeared. Rick went to see his physician and he was diagnosed as HIV positive. His doctor explained the complications of his situation, putting tremendous emphasis on how different his lifestyle would have to be if he intended to live much longer.

Rick entered a rehab clinic equipped to treat him for his drug and alcohol dependencies, but his health had already declined to an extreme degree, and he began to appear quite sick. One month after his release, his health took another hit when he came down with the flu and lost over thirty pounds. He looked like a skeleton and his eyes began to sink in. It was apparent that Rick had a serious illness, and soon even hookers were unwilling to be intimate with him. Rick was frantic. He started relying on cocaine, alcohol, and tobacco again, but nothing could replace the release he desired through sex.

One of Rick's long time friends suggested he work with The Witnessing Technique, so he made an appointment. He was in good spirits when he arrived, but he was very fidgety, and he had the shakes. After a lot of nervous joking around, he expressed that his greatest fear at the time was of being sexually deprived. Rick was guided to close his eyes and allow his fear to form into an image, and the vision of a trembling skeleton appeared. It was shaking violently, and the area where his penis would have been was gushing with blood. Rick watched the image for a while and commented that the only life the skeleton had was in his penis, which symbolized that sex ran his life.

Rick sat quietly for a moment, and then he commented that he had always been terrified of how empty his life felt before he started singing on stage, having sex, and taking drugs. He admitted that the lifestyle he had chosen may not have been fulfilling him after all; it had merely been an escape from his pain. Rick was guided to allow his "old empty pain" to form into an image, and the vision of a man screaming with a very large, wide-open mouth appeared. The image never took a breath. It only kept screaming, as if the scream had been held in for so long it had no end.

Rick sat with the image for a while and found it to be quite a euphoric feeling in the end. As his pain transformed through the screaming image, he could feel sexual tension in his body relax and release. After fifteen minutes of watching *the scream*, Rick opened his eyes and shared that he felt as though he had just let go of thirty years of suppressed fear and pain.

Instead of being released through a climax, his sexual energy had trans-formed inside of his body and caused a euphoria he described as "beyond

words." Rick was shocked to discover that his inner reality held more fulfillment for him than any outer experience he had ever encountered.

*We can use our sexual energy in three ways. We can release it through climax,
suppress it with will-power, or transform it with The Witnessing Technique.
When sexual energy is transformed, it will ignite the indescribable bliss of Pure
Consciousness within. Sexual energy is Life Force. We can use it to give birth to
a higher state of consciousness within ourselves, just as Rick did.*

At Rick's next appointment, he was happy to report that each time he
watched the screaming face, he felt much more comfortable in his body.
His sleep had improved, and his disturbance over sexual abstinence was
also diminishing. His sexual desires had toned down to such a degree that
he was finally able to fall asleep without ejaculating first. He still craved
sex, but he no longer felt as though he would explode without it. The
image of the shaking skeleton occurred less and less during his witnessing
practices and the screaming face was "almost all screamed out," as Rick
put it.

Rick was astonished by how simple the technique was and how quickly
he saw transformation occur. He commented that if he had only known
how to look within and transform his pain long ago, he might have a much
healthier body at that moment. Rick had a lot of concern over what was
happening to his body, because it was dwindling quickly, and he feared that
death was near. He allowed this fear to form into an image, and the vision
of an empty broken-down house in the middle of a desert appeared. It had
been abandoned, and the wind was blowing through cracked, brittle, paint-
chipped window shutters that had torn away from their hinges. Everything
in the image was a sallow, yellow-gray, but what affected him the most was
that it was empty, with no one around who cared. Rick said he felt just like
the house. He was all alone and deprived of the love and caring for which
he yearned. In fact, he had felt abandoned, alone, deprived, empty, and
afraid of loss his entire life. He believed that no one would care about him
no matter what was happening to him.

Once Rick had reached a neutral feeling about the broken-down house, he was able to identify with his *Witnessing Self* and experience a deep peacefulness. As he continued to practice the technique, he established a sense of tranquility that was ever present.

As is often the case when death is near, Rick plunged into his inner reality more deeply than most, eager to find a sense of security in his remaining days. During his last few sessions, Rick playfully reminisced about his life, pointing out that he had known the extremes of physical bliss, but was fortunate enough to experience a feeling that he could only describe as "inner bliss."

Rick left his body three months later. He wrote in his own eulogy that he would die a happy man who had finally found a true sense of peace and fulfillment deep within, which he had longed for all his life.

Witnessing: A Path to Overcome
Addiction to the Past

Carla was a very open girl who rarely stopped talking unless she was asleep. She spoke during movies and television shows, at funerals during the ceremony, at weddings during the vows, at events over the presenters, and at her place of worship over the Cleric.

What Carla's friends complained about the most, however, was that her favorite topic of conversation was her painful past. No matter how patient, polite, or attentive people were, Carla was insatiable. If anyone offered verbal consolation, she would burst into tears and complain that they were not listening to her. A new acquaintance who felt true compassion for Carla, suggested The Witnessing Technique, so she made an appointment right away.

Carla arrived for her session thirty minutes early, speaking non-stop on her cell phone for all to hear while she waited. When her session began, Carla made it clear right up front that she felt it would be imperative to express every detail of just how horrific and depressing her life had been, starting from the day she was born. Because this was the pattern Carla needed to rise above the most, she was gently told that she would be led into something that would feel even better than that. Carla was shocked. She had never realized how much she enjoyed complaining about her past.

The most painful feeling that Carla experienced in her everyday life was emotional abandonment. When she was guided to allow her feelings to form into an image, however, she was unable to do so, because she did not trust that anyone would understand her unless she had divulged the full history of her painful past. Unwilling to proceed any further with the technique, Carla was invited to share the core pain that was troubling her, while paying close attention to how her body responded as she expressed herself. If her body became tense or uncomfortable, she was instructed to stop.

Carla ignored these prerequisites and embarked upon her painful history in the old habitual way, becoming extremely animated and dramatic immediately. She went into fits of weeping, yelling, and heavy breathing as she shared the same painful story that she must had shared thousands of times before. Her mind had convinced her that speaking about it would calm her down. Instead, she became more riled up as the intimate details of her story were revealed. She was working herself into a frenzy over something her brother had said to her thirty-six years ago.

Carla was tenderly reminded that she was to stay in touch with her body while she expressed herself, so she closed her eyes, tuned into her body, and shared that her shoulders had caved in, her neck had grown tight, her stomach and throat had seized up, her head had begun to pound, and she could feel the beginning of a migraine. She was then invited to relax and focus on her breath as it moved in and out. After a few moments,

Carla shared that her shoulders had opened and relaxed, her head had cooled down and stopped pounding, and the acidy feeling in her stomach had dissipated.

She was then given the option to move toward a gentle transformation of her pain that would save her body from any further stress, and her response was, "But I am not finished yet." Then she launched right back into a vicious verbal account of her brother. After a few moments she was reminded once again to pay close attention to her body. She let out a groan and admitted that she could feel her head getting hot and turning red. She could feel the veins popping out in her forehead, and her stomach was turning acidy and tense. *This is one example of how people become sick. They avoid what their body is telling them, and it breaks down.* Eventually, Carla realized that whenever she complained about the past, her entire being felt weak, sick, heavy, tense, and fiery. The worse she felt, the more she wanted to blame her brother for her pain. When Carla brought herself into the moment with her own breath, she felt light and peaceful again.

Once Carla's body had recuperated, she was asked if she saw herself as her painful past and her response was, "Yes, I guess so. What else would I be if I am not my past?" Carla was then very gently asked if she wanted everyone to perceive her as a victim. She immediately stood up and screamed, "I am NOT a victim!" Carla was then guided to question what impression she thought she was giving to people if her favorite topic of conversation was about how victimized she had been in the past and how much the past still hurts her.

This might sound harsh to those who are also in so much pain they cannot stop talking about their past, but please understand that the kindest thing you can do for yourself and others is to detach from the drama and move into The Witnessing Technique. Complaining will only make the pain grow.

When Carla finally allowed her feelings to form into an image, the vision of a small baby crying all alone in a crib appeared. She watched as the baby continued to cry louder and louder for over seven minutes in her imagination. (*When pain is expressed through the image, it will dissipate and transform. This is a healthy avenue of expression.*) When the image of the crying baby had lost its emotional charge for Carla, she was finally able to leave the painful abandoned feelings with the baby and identify with the aspect of her consciousness that was able to observe the image. Once Carla identified with her *Witnessing Self*, she immediately felt empowered. She was clear that she was not the baby; she was the observer of the baby and its pain. As the *witness*, she was separate from the image and the suffering it represented.

Carla was then asked if given the choice to identify with her *Witnessing Self* or with the crying baby, which one she would choose. She laughed and said, "Well, of course, my *Witnessing Self*." Carla then recognized that for most of her life she had been choosing to identify with her "helpless victim" programming, and she felt awakened by the new option she had available to her.

Because Carla's mind had been addicted to extremes for so long; along with constantly talking and constantly seeking outside attention, when she allowed a pause in this momentum, her mind suddenly stopped. She reported that after her first full day of practicing The Witnessing Technique, she felt physically sick when she thought of speaking about her past. In fact, she did not have the urge to speak at all for three days, and she thought she was losing her mind. She was petrified, because it was so different from what she was used to.

Carla *was* losing her mind in a manner of speaking, because she was rising above the programming in her mind. For those who have lived in their mind in extremes, as Carla did, the transition from constant chatter to silence is a jolt to the system. Similar to waking up from a nightmare, they will feel unsteady and frightened for a short while. The talkative person cuts out half of their programming just by becoming silent. Also, the mind and the past are synonymous. They go together. When the mind is still, the past has no way of entering. As Carla continued to *witness* her image, she felt lighter, happier and freer each day. She was finally allowing her true self to come forth by identifying with Pure Consciousness.

When Carla arrived for her third session she was a different person, overflowing with gratitude after realizing how much she had to celebrate. Carla had recognized, as if for the first time, that she was a talented musician, she lived in a beautiful home, she had a gift with animals, she was a great decorator, and she had enough wealth to do anything she wanted. Carla was elated to finally experience happiness about her life. She had never realized that living in the past negated her life in the moment.

This radical shift might appear unbelievable to most, but the more radical the behavior, often the more radical the shift will be. There was a conscious part of Carla that was ready to let go of her pain, even though her mind was still attached to it. The healthier part of our consciousness will always succeed when The Witnessing Technique is applied. No longer engrossed in the hurtful events from her past, Carla continues to celebrate the blessings of each new day. Every moment spent as the *witness* highlights her good fortune.

Witnessing: A Path to Overcome
Addiction to Drama

Martha was in an extremely abusive relationship with a man named Darren, who was an alcoholic, drug abuser, sex addict, and chain smoker. During Martha's pregnancy, she discovered that Darren was having an affair with her cousin, her sister, and her aunt. Martha was afraid to leave Darren, because she believed she needed his support. He had financial means, and Martha had given up her job to be with him and have his baby.

Martha's life had played out like a soap opera since she was a child. Her parents were alcoholics, and there had been a lot of inner family sexual indiscretion happening that "shocked the neighbors," as Martha put it. Without something extraordinarily scandalous happening in Martha's life, she felt alone and unimportant. The more painful and dramatic her life became, the more she had to talk about and worry about and work through, which seemed to give her a sense of purpose.

When Martha and Darren first met, Martha was doing well for herself. No one could believe that she would become involved with someone as notoriously abusive as Darren. According to their mental programming, however, it was a perfect match. She was a victim, and he was an abuser, and they were both addicted to drama. *More often than not, the chemistry couples experience in the beginning of a relationship is based on programming of this sort.*

While Martha was pregnant, she consulted her lawyer about leaving Darren. Her lawyer gave her good legal advice and also suggested that she seek emotional support. Martha agreed and made an appointment to work with The Witnessing Technique the next day.

When Martha arrived she was frantic. Her car had been broken into, and many of her new purchases for the baby had been taken. Her nylons were ripped because she had tripped over her sprinkler system at home, and she had a headache from banging her head into her bathroom mirror in the middle of the night. After Martha had settled down, she recounted explicitly, and in detail, numerous instances of daily drama. The intricate turmoil of her relationships seemed to intoxicate her. She needed desperately for someone to acknowledge her pain and understand how much she was hurting. When others did not believe the drama of her life, she became distraught and exasperated when she tried to prove it to them.

After Martha had shared her most recent discovery of finding her sister and aunt in bed with Darren at the same time, she expressed that the most painful emotion she had experienced in her relationships with others was the feeling of being worthless and stupid. Martha closed her eyes and allowed these feelings to take the form of an image, and the vision of a cartoon figure appeared that resembled a disheveled Daffy Duck. It marched around in circles, flapping its wings and squawking with its head down. As long as the wings were flapping, the bird could focus on the chaotic movement of its feathers and avoid the feelings of shame and worthlessness.

Martha was guided to connect with the aspect of her consciousness that was able to observe the duck. Once she had identified with her *Witnessing Self*, she was able to rise above the pain the duck symbolized. She realized that the image only *represented a belief* that she was worthless and stupid. Her image did not represent her *true self* at all.

When Martha returned for her second session she was more present, but still frantic about the happenings of her day. When she closed her eyes and allowed her feelings to form into an image, the vision of a female slave tied to a pillar with her clothes half ripped off appeared. Martha watched the image and expressed that the slave had been raped and beaten while everyone stood around watching. She wailed for help, but the onlookers appeared uninterested and bored. No one seemed to care.

The image of the slave expressed the hopelessness Martha experienced in her life. She believed that someone had to come to her rescue in order for her life to improve. Her happiness and worth were always in someone else's hands. As long as no one came to rescue her, she was convinced that she was unlovable; which was the core fear around which her personality was formed. Her mind concluded that she would be trapped in her current abusive situation forever, because life was not going to get any better no matter what *she* did. The programming in Martha's mind portrayed her as a perpetual victim who would be forever humiliated, abused, and abandoned.

Martha reached a neutral feeling about the slave by watching her scream for over five minutes in her mind. When she was finally able to detach and *witness* the image, she was once again relieved to discover that the character only represented programming in her mind. Feeling victimized, helpless, unloved, and unwanted, did not have to be her reality any longer.

When Martha was asked to describe her experience as the *witness*, her face became radiant and tears began flowing down her cheeks. As the *witness*, she saw herself as an emanation of love, no longer having to wait for love from the outer world. She was elated by this discovery, and she felt excited about expanding on her *true essence*. She agreed to practice identifying with her Witnessing Self throughout the week.

On Martha's next visit she appeared much more centered and confident. She spoke about leaving Darren and getting her life back into balance on her own. She felt confident that no matter what a split would put her through, it would be less dramatic and less abusive than staying with Darren. During this session, the image of the slave appeared again and Martha was able to observe the "perpetual martyr" aspect of her personality and choose not to identify with her painful feelings of being victimized.

Even with all these insights, however, Martha still felt a strong desire to condemn those who betrayed her by telling dramatic stories. She understood that each time she shared her passionate accounts of her abuse, her programming would strengthen, but she simply could not help herself.

Gossiping about her pain had become an addiction itself. She had a particularly difficult time trying not to condemn Darren. Eventually she understood that the more she condemned him, the stronger her attraction would be to him, as her mind would seek resolution from him.

When a victim wants the abuser to pay for his or her mistakes or make it up, this keeps the victim attached to the abuser and to the pain. Remember, pain arises from our ego and its attachments, not from the other person. If Martha had not met Darren, she simply would have attracted a different abuser. Even if the abuser is punished or apologizes, it will not heal the pain involved with the abuse. Healing is an inside job. We must rise above the patterns that attracted our trauma in the first place to feel free from the pain and to create healthy unions in the future.

When Martha was able to identify with her *Witnessing Self,* she realized that the less emotional and dramatic she became about everything, the easier it was to remain aware, clear, and strong. When she identified with her pain, the programming took a hold of her mercilessly, and she would become the helpless, abused slave in her image, waiting for someone to take pity on her and rescue her.

Martha practiced The Witnessing Technique diligently for the next few months. Darren was put into a rehab program, because he had beaten one of his lovers while he was high on crack cocaine. Instead of becoming involved with condemning Darren or telling everyone about it, Martha was able to focus her energy positively and establish a new home for herself where she felt safe and strong. Darren did not want anything to do with Martha or the child, so she had the child on her own and started a new life intent on having no drama or victimization. Martha was able to find a good job and married a very loving and kind man two years later.

Choosing an abusive partner is quite common for those who have been programmed to believe they are worthless. Martha's programming caused her to gravitate toward someone who appeared to be of less worth, according to her own standards, in hopes that this "even less significant" person would love her. Inevitably, this type of choice backfires, because the less self-esteem a person has, often the more abusive they become. When an individual is controlled by the mind, this type of destructive scenario frequently occurs.

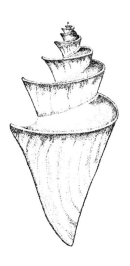

CHAPTER 7

Compulsive Thoughts and Emotions

Introduction

Strong irresistible impulses,
which repeat themselves in a relentless cycle,
often leading to destructive, addictive,
or habitual behavior.

OMPULSIVE INDIVIDUALS IDENTIFY WITH THE MIND and its programming to such an extreme degree that they become helplessly
consumed by impulses which determine their actions. Every core fear
will structure the mind to depend upon one specific emotional-reaction as
the common response to any stressful situation in life. For example, the core
fear of being unimportant will compel an individual to rely on anger as their
common response to distress. No matter what occurs, this person will seek
out a reason to be angry. The core fear of having no purpose will compel an
individual to rely on blame. The core fear of being unsafe will cause an individual to rely on panic. The ability to respond intelligently or appropriately

- 133 -

is overshadowed by these programmed reactions, upon which the mind depends time and time again.

Compulsive Behavior

Overwhelming thoughts and emotions often lead a compulsive mind to crave immediate gratification and force an individual to act on desires in an irrational way. The compulsive liar believes his lie is *required*. The compulsive eater is *possessed* by their desire for food. The compulsive gambler will feel *besieged* by their desire to risk.

The mind yearns to be active or engaged. If it becomes bored, stressed, or is uninvolved with other tasks, the compulsive imprint is activated. In extreme cases, an individual may have compulsive thoughts which lead to compulsive crimes.

All compulsive behavior stems from the programming in the mind. To be free from this imbalance, we must rise above the mind and identify with the aspect of our consciousness that is innately free from all destructive programming.

Witnessing: A Path to Overcome

Extroverted Compulsive Rage

David was a very successful attorney with a loving wife, four children, and two mistresses. Working cases in New York, Chicago, and Boston allowed him the opportunity to have lovers in each city. When David spent time at his main office in New York, he often found himself angry and irritated with his employees. He would yell at members of his staff in front of their co-workers until they broke down in tears or a fight ensued. Most of his employees left the office disgraced and trembling each night.

At home, David was hostile with his small children and his wife. If the dinner was not to his liking, he would scream at his wife and humiliate her in front of the children. If the children started to cry, David would whisk them into their rooms and reprimand them severely.

One day when David was in Chicago working on a big case, his Chicago mistress called to inform him that she was pregnant. David was livid. He exploded out of the office, arrived at her apartment with a baseball bat in his hand, and smashed lamps and flower arrangements in a rage. When he lifted the bat ready to hit his mistress, he noticed a uniformed officer standing in the doorway. The police officer took a report and suggested David stay away from his mistress.

News of this incident reached his wife, who threatened to file for a divorce unless he received counseling for his compulsive anger and infidelity. David did not want to lose his family, so he agreed. He was about to begin some work in Los Angeles, so his sister suggested The Witnessing Technique and called ahead to set up his appointment.

When David arrived, his energy was overly self-confident and dominant. He was confrontational at first, wanting to make it clear that he was the one in charge. When David was asked to get in touch with the emotion with which he had the most difficulty, he replied that he had no difficulty with any emotions. He went on to say that he had no problems at all, and that the world was just filled with imbeciles who he had to keep in line. David continued in this fashion for fifty-five minutes, unwilling to admit any emotion and reluctant to becoming vulnerable in any way. What he expressed was acknowledged, and another appointment was set up.

This is common behavior for individuals who have a core fear of not being in control. Their mind will rely upon domination—usually enforced through rage—as the common response to stress. Their mental programming creates a personality that feels superior to others as a defense against feeling vulnerable or needing anyone. As our sessions continued, David admitted that he consciously intended to harm others in a manner they would never forget, before they had a chance to harm or betray him. He felt it was important to keep people intimidated with his rage, so they would think twice about crossing him. David's programming had convinced him that terrorizing others was the best response to any stressful situation in life.

On David's fifth session he appeared upset. With a broken voice, he confided that his youngest son had told him that he hated him. This incident brought up fear that he would be rejected, and eventually abandoned, by his son. David was invited to allow his feelings to form into an image in his mind. He followed along with the directions as if he were a changed man and closed his eyes. The vision that appeared for him was a small boy standing outside of a building. The child had a knapsack on his back and a brown bag lunch clutched in his tiny hand. David described him as tenderly as he had ever spoken. He named the boy in his image "Johnny" and went on to explain how broken-hearted the boy looked. Johnny was waiting for someone to come and pick him up, but as long as he waited, no one arrived. He felt abandoned and rejected.

David opened his eyes and eventually shared that the image reminded him of his childhood. When his father died, David's mother left him with his grandmother in order to appease a new boyfriend who did not want David around. One day his mother promised to meet him in front of a dime store so they could spend the day together. David was so excited that he got up before the sun rose to prepare. He made his mother and himself a brown bag lunch and ran outside ready for her by 6:00 a.m. David waited for her all day long, but she never arrived. He did not return home until it was dark, still holding hope in his heart that his mother would want to see him again one day.

David's mother did not call to apologize or explain, however, she did contact him a few months later to set up another meeting and promised to show up. David jumped out of bed with new-found hope and rushed off to meet her in front of the dime store. Once again he waited all day and half way into the night, but his mother did not appear. David's heart was shattered again. This same sort of event occurred every two to three months over a two year period, but David never saw his mother again. Finally, he refused to take her calls.

After this point, whenever David felt vulnerable to the pain of being rejected, forgotten, or betrayed, he would fly into a rage. This was his way of warning people not to disappoint him. The more he cared about an individual, the more he *tried* to bring out the worst in them, in an attempt to find reasons not to love them. Then he could discard them more easily and never encounter the pain of missing them. However, no matter how many people he terrorized with his rage, the pain of his mother's abandonment did not go away, and people still betrayed him, even though they feared him. His programming was not giving him a real solution to his pain.

David was guided to watch the image of Johnny while the boy expressed his fear of being rejected and abandoned. The small child remained vulnerable and innocent, hoping his mother would cherish him as much as he cherished her one day. He never stopped loving her. In fact, he opened his heart more, hoping she would feel his love and be drawn to his energy.

As David watched the eternally loving image of the boy, he became angry. He was guided to allow his new emotion to form into another image, and a rock figure with a club in his hand appeared. He named the figure "Rocky" and went on to describe how much Rocky loved the boy. Rocky's sole purpose was to protect Johnny by standing in front of him, clubbing anyone who came close. Rocky saw everyone else as the enemy. He trusted no one and felt complete loyalty to the child he guarded. Johnny was the only *real* being. Everyone else had no heart or soul, so Rocky had full permission, without conscience, to attack or kill those who threatened the little boy and his precious vulnerability. *Rocky symbolized the programming in David's mind that caused him to close off to everyone in order to protect his sensitive, child-like heart.*

After five minutes of watching Rocky clobber everyone in the vicinity, David was guided to connect with the aspect of his consciousness that was able to observe the image of Rocky. Once he had identified with his *Witnessing Self*, his aggressive body language melted, and he sat back into his seat very relaxed. He was silent for quite a while, then he shared that to his surprise, he felt significantly more powerful as the *witness* than he did when he identified with the tough character of Rocky. This new perspective felt promising to David, so he agreed to continue *witnessing* the image throughout the week. David left the appointment that day, and for the first time he smiled and said thank you. His movements were gentle and calm. The true sensitivity of his nature was beginning to shine through.

On David's eighth session, he shared a mental battle he was having over choosing anger to gain respect during confrontations at work. He still believed there was a place for intimidating others in business. David was asked if he felt people truly respected him, or if he thought they might be unsettled by his aggressive tactics and inspired to work out of fear. David laughed an uncomfortable laugh and looked away. He wanted to believe that people respected him, but deep down he knew that he was more feared than admired. He admitted that it was possible he would end up like *Scrooge* from, "A Christmas Carol," all alone in his dying days, with people waiting around to distribute his wealth.

In an attempt to assist David in moving beyond his compulsive anger, he was guided to look within and discover why his *Witnessing Self* (his ego-less self) felt so much more powerful than the image of Rocky (his ego-programming.) He closed his eyes, and when he finally spoke, his voice was deeper than usual and very peaceful. David shared that he experienced his *Witnessing Self* as pure compassion. He saw no danger in exuding compassion around others, because it only made him more powerful, calm, and aware. His *Witnessing Self* also felt much more capable of protecting his "inner child" than the image of Rocky did, so he had no reason to be defensive or angry as a protective measure. David finally realized that he could be powerful and protected without the use of force.

After three months of intensive transformation, David went home, apologized to his wife for his previous behavior, and reconnected with his children in a new way. Instead of trying to intimidate or force them to love and respect him, he began to show love and respect to his family. This new choice worked brilliantly, and David's family life improved tremendously.

As he continued to practice The Witnessing Technique on his own, David found it necessary to change his line of work. He now owns a string of children's toy stores and helps in the design of the toy line he is developing. David made his family his main focus, and he is a much happier man. *He has opened his heart, and he is willing to love again, which makes it impossible to be violent with those he cares about.*

Now that David is in touch with how much he loves and appreciates his wife, he no longer finds the need for mistresses or sexual affairs. His mistress in Chicago had a miscarriage, and David paid for her medical expenses and said goodbye. David still has a gruff manner about him and more programming to rise above, but his previously piercing, angry eyes have become like a small child's. They are innocent, open, and loving.

Anger is a very powerful emotion. When it is faced, it can transform a person's life in many positive ways. Our emotions are gifts that can help us discover our deepest programming. In most cases, people find that their anger is part of a program that keeps them from love as a protective measure. Compulsive anger is usually a sign that a significant shift in perspective is necessary.

Witnessing: A Path to Overcome

Introverted Compulsive Rage

Tommy was a mild-mannered business man who had been married for ten years. When he spent time with his wife, however, he found himself experiencing such extreme levels of internal rage that he began to fear he might lose his control and do something out of character. His rage had become so prevalent that it was affecting his health, musculature, and ability to focus.

On Tommy's wife's birthday, he surprised her with the dream car that she had always wanted by wrapping it in a red bow and putting twelve long-stemmed red roses in the front seat. When Tommy's wife discovered the car, her only comment was that she did not like the tires he had chosen. Then she stomped back into the house and slammed the door. Tommy took the car back and had her preferred tires put on, but when he arrived home, his wife complained that he had not washed it again before bringing it to her as a gift. Tommy had been faced with situations of this sort for nine years before he began to snap. As his anger grew, he started feeling an inner desire to kill his wife, which is quite common when anger is suppressed.

Tommy believed that suppressing his anger would be the best choice, because he feared that his wife would only behave more atrociously if he did express it. As his rage grew, however, he found himself losing his temper over the slightest things. If the wind blew his hair across his face, he felt ready to scream. If he missed a green light on the way to work, he wanted to shoot the light.

When Tommy took his wife on trips, he would turn violently ill for no apparent reason and often end up in the hospital. He also began having "accidents." He would get into fender benders, rip the jacket of a new Armani suit, drop his day planner in a sink full of water and shaving crème, etc. He broke his leg, sprained his ankle, and burned his hand while he was making his wife dinner. He cut himself badly while shaving almost every week, and he frequently threw his back out so severely that he could hardly move. These injuries would occur within one hour of having an incident with his wife. He also started losing important things, such as his cell phone, his wallet, his car keys, and his work assignments. His compulsive rage showed itself in many ways. Even though he did not take it out on his wife, he was taking it out on himself daily.

One day Tommy's wife pushed him beyond his limits, and he yelled at her, which was quite out of character for him. His wife was so outraged that she threw all the china in the kitchen at him and destroyed the entire set, which happened to be Tommy's mother's original set from her wedding day. After that, Tommy began praying daily for his wife to die or find another man and leave him so he could be free. He often fantasized about sexy young women who would love him and be appreciative of him as a distraction from his grief, but his core fear of being *disturbed* would not allow him to take outward action to make any changes to alleviate his pain. After noticing the increasingly detached and ineffectual behavior of Tommy at work, a business associate suggested he begin working with The Witnessing Technique, so he made an appointment that day.

When Tommy arrived for his session he expressed his pain very politely, all the while clenching his fists and grinding his teeth. When Tommy was guided to allow his rage to emerge as an image, the ominous figure of Darth Vader appeared. Tommy felt suddenly empowered as he watched the character engage his light-saber and defeat his wife with a single blow. Darth went on to obliterate the room he was in as he slashed everything up in sight.

After a few minutes, Tommy opened his eyes to express concern over how violent the image had been. He was working out his repressed emotions in a healthy way, so he was encouraged to continue to allow the image complete freedom to vent its rage in whatever manner came forth naturally from the character.

Tommy closed his eyes again and continued to allow Darth all the violence and vengeance he needed in his mind for over twelve minutes. When he finally opened his eyes, his body was relaxed and his face had a light glow about it. Now that his rage had been neutralized, Tommy was guided to connect with the aspect of his consciousness that was able to observe the image. He identified with his *Witnessing Self* easily, surprised to discover that as the *witness*, he felt much more omnipotent than his dominating Darth Vader character. Tommy was excited to continue with the technique on his own during the week. He left the office with a spring in his step and a genuine smile on his face.

When Tommy arrived for his next session, he was very animated as he expressed the success he had experienced moving through life as the *witness* for one week. He had neither injured himself nor had he lost or destroyed anything. Tommy was also much less angry around his wife. However, he had a new concern. Why had he allowed his wife to treat him with such disrespect in the first place?

Tommy was guided to close his eyes and allow the feeling of being disrespected to form into an image, and the vision of a Slave Horse appeared. The horse had a painful harness around his mouth and throat, and he was tightly tied up to a stall, making it impossible for him to move even one inch. The horse felt trapped, constrained, controlled, abused, and unhappy. It did not feel loved or cared for at all.

Tommy was guided to allow the horse to express its pain until he felt neutral about the image. Once that had been accomplished, he was invited to identify with his *Witnessing Self* and view the Slave Horse as a program in his mind. *According to Tommy's ego, his own happiness was dependent on being able to please others.* If he was unable to please his wife, he felt trapped in his pain, unable to move forward in any direction safely. This image brought up his core fear of being *disturbed*. The more disturbed he became, the more hopelessness built in his mind. The only path his ego would allow to alleviate his disturbed feelings, was to find a way to please his wife. Yet, even if he tried his best, he never had any guarantee that his wife would agree to be pleased. When he failed at pleasing her, he became angry. Consequently, Tommy was left feeling like a slave to her emotions.

Tommy left on a three week vacation with his wife the weekend after his second session and agreed to identify with his *Witnessing Self* by rising above the "Slave Horse" programming each morning before he began the day. When Tommy returned, he reported that he had not become ill on his trip for the first time in five years. His anger no longer had the ability to overpower him and cause him to hurt himself. He also discovered that he was beginning to interact with his wife as the strong, confident man he wanted to be, instead of a wimpy victim who she crushed with criticism. His wife began showing Tommy much more respect and appreciation once this shift occurred, and their relationship continues to improve as his *Witnessing Self* strengthens.

The Witnessing Technique is not only experienced by the individuals practicing the technique, but also by everyone who crosses their path. Those practicing will become radiant with freedom from their previous burden, and people close to them will feel lighter and happier in their presence.

Witnessing: A Path to Overcome

Compulsive Jealousy

Barry was a busy CPA who often had late meetings and worked weekends in the office. His wife Linda trusted him at first, but when his business expanded, she feared that his lack of attentiveness meant he was interested in someone else. As her insecurities heightened, she would drill Barry about his day and demand to know where he had been and with whom. Many times she would call his secretary or business partner to confirm his story. If Barry arrived home a few minutes later than usual, Linda would attack him or start crying, trying to illicit sympathy for her jealousy and loneliness.

Barry was accommodating at first, keeping in mind that Linda's first husband had been unfaithful. However, it hurt him that she did not trust him, and the more she tried to monitor and control his time, the more he wanted to escape. As conflict increased, Barry began considering a divorce. Linda was desperate to have him stay, but she felt she was right. She constantly complained to her friends about Barry, until one friend suggested that she work on her own fears and stop expecting Barry to live his life according to her insecurities. Linda was shocked. She had never considered what she was asking Barry to do. Her friend also recommended The Witnessing Technique, so she made an appointment right away.

When Linda arrived, she expressed her fears and jealousies, emphasizing that when Barry would not come home on time, his behavior made her feel "not good enough." Linda was guided to close her eyes and allow her fear to form into an image, and the vision of a Police Officer with a whistle and ticket pad appeared in her mind. He had a sly arrogant look on his face, as if he were hoping for the chance to catch a "bad guy."

When Linda imagined Barry walking in the door late, she saw the image of the Police Officer whip out his ticket pad, ready to write Barry a citation without any provocation. Barry was innocent, however, so Linda's mind made up reasons to punish and condemn him.

When Linda was guided to connect with the aspect of her consciousness that was able to observe the image of the Police Officer, she understood that her fears were self-generated and that Barry was an honest man. As Linda continued to *witness* her mind, she found that her Police Officer programming appeared around friends and family as well. Her fear of not being good enough created disharmony with every relationship she had.

Determined to improve her life, Linda practiced the technique diligently and made a commitment to look for the good in herself and others, which was the opposite of the programming in her mind. Within a few weeks she was seeing the world in a new light, and she felt more confident about herself with each passing day. From this new perspective, she was able to comment on those things she loved about Barry, instead of tearing him down. Soon he felt he had the woman with whom he had fallen in love back again. He stopped talking about divorce and started coming home earlier and more often.

Both Barry and Linda practice The Witnessing Technique on their own throughout the day and can now laugh about the characters that their minds impose on them when they are unaware and fearful. Whenever Linda becomes suspicious or condemning, Barry laughs and says, "Yes, Officer." His serious-kidding shakes Linda into her senses, and they can both have a good giggle.

Witnessing: A Path to Overcome

Compulsive Lying

Dick wanted to move to Hollywood to become an actor. His big brother Dave arranged for him to live in a guest house behind his wealthy fraternity brother, Colin, who had a home in the Hollywood Hills. When Dick arrived on the property, he immediately wanted to own the spectacular estate, and he began telling people that it was his. "Fake it until you make it," was his motto.

Dick had very little luck in the movie industry, but he was able to fill in as an extra on a few "B" films, so he told people that he was a working actor. He made up a fictitious resume and sent it out to agents and managers, but no one seemed interested. Dick was discouraged. He wanted everything to happen immediately so he could buy a big house and impress a lot of people.

Shortly after Dick moved in, Colin went on a business trip for one week, leaving Dick in charge of the house. The moment he was out the door, Dick went into Colin's room and scrounged together over two thousand dollars. Then he went directly into Colin's vintage car garage, (which was specifically off limits) and hopped into the most valuable car in the collection. Burning rubber off the property, Dick sped right to his favorite bar on Sunset Boulevard and bought a round of drinks for everyone. Then he stood on a table and informed the group that he had just landed a big part in a movie with Tom Cruise. His audience seemed interested, and Dick was finally getting the attention he craved.

Dick took Shelley, his cocktail waitress, up to Colin's house so he could romance her in Colin's master bedroom, which had a 180 degree view of the city. He drove her home the next day in a different vintage car and told her he had a big meeting with Tom Cruise to go over scripts that afternoon. Shelley was quite excited by Dick's impressive display, so she made herself available to him every night that week.

When Colin was about to arrive back home, Dick told Shelley he would be on location in Japan filming his movie for a few months, but that he would call her the minute he arrived back in town. Then Dick telephoned the police to report that someone had broken into Colin's house. He made it look as if a forced entry had occurred, and he disheveled Colin's room so it would appear that someone had frantically gone through all his belongings.

When Colin arrived home he was suspicious. He noticed many of the vintage cars were dirty and parked in the wrong spaces. He questioned Dick, who suggested that the thief had also taken the cars out for a spin. He went on to elaborate that he had heard about the same type of burglary before many times. Colin had not trusted Dick very much from the beginning, and the police were suspicious as well.

Dick ran into Shelley by accident a few months later, so they sat down for coffee. Dick told Shelley that he had just purchased a new house, and that his cash and credit were tied up in escrow. He wondered if she would loan him one thousand dollars until his cash flow situation changed. Shelley agreed and wrote him a check. Dick had no intention of re-paying Shelley, but she tracked him down a few weeks later by incessantly calling his cell phone. Dick finally agreed to meet her and wrote her a check for fifteen hundred dollars, insisting on paying her interest. When Shelley went to his bank, however, she discovered that Dick's account had been closed. In fury, Shelly drove up to the Hollywood Hills house, and Colin answered the door. Shelley and Colin had a long talk, but when Colin confronted Dick with the truth, he denied everything. Colin finally had Dick's brother intervene, and Dick agreed to go into counseling for his compulsive lying.

When Dick showed up for his session he was charismatic, likable, and as innocent looking as a young man could be. One would never suspect that he was one step away from becoming a professional con artist. Dick spent most of his time making jokes and telling elaborate "stories" about his success, making it very clear that he was not ready to face the truth. He left the session convinced that he had made an impressive show and that everything would be smoothed over once word of his perfect character got back to his brother Dave.

When Dick arrived for his next session, he was angry, because he had been caught making fake ID's, and charges were being pressed against him. He was guided to allow his anger to form into an image, and the vision of a frantic jailbird in an old black and white striped prison uniform appeared. The image resembled a trickster out of a Charlie Chaplin movie with a ball and chain around his ankle. The character expressed his rage by pulling harder and harder on the ball until flames shot out of his temples. Dick said he hated the character because he was "a big stupid mistake." He was silent for a while, and when he opened his eyes, he suggested that we move on to something else. When he was asked why he wanted to change the subject, Dick said that it was no big deal, but then he muttered under his breath that *he was a big mistake.*

Eventually he confided that his conception was unplanned, and that his parents did not want him. Dick displayed a lot of sadness as he recalled this memory and finished his story by sharing that no matter how hard he tried, he would *never be enough* to make his mother happy that he existed. He believed that he would have to be superhuman in order to be accepted in her life.

Dick was guided to allow his sadness to form into an image, and the vision of a Pinocchio Doll appeared. It could talk and it appeared "real," but it was actually half doll-half boy. The real part of him was sad, and the doll part of him had a happy face. The image would dance and smile and do all sorts of tricks, but all the while the doll was crying inside.

Dick was guided to connect with the aspect of his consciousness that was able to observe the image. Once he had identified with his *Witnessing Self,* he was able to detach from the idea that he was not enough. As the *witness*, he saw through the illusion that he would have to lie about who he was in order to impress others. However, he was still attached to the idea that he was a mistake.

Dick was invited to close his eyes and allow the feeling of being a mistake to form into an image, and the vision of Dick as a baby appeared in his mind. Once he had identified with his *Witnessing Self,* he realized that the tiny baby that had been created by "mistake," (according to his mother), was perfect. He did not appear to be a mistake at all. As the *witness*, Dick saw clearly that the child was wanted, necessary, and loved. In fact, he was quite impressed by the child's precious energy.

The revelations of this session impacted Dick so profoundly that he agreed to *witness* his images throughout the week. True to his word, he arrived for his following session with a much deeper connection to his *Witnessing Self.* As he continued to look within and apply the technique, his consciousness evolved and raised his level of self-confidence and personal power very quickly. Within one month of this transformation, Dick admitted his interest in acting had begun when one of his girlfriends professed her infatuation with Tom Cruise. His real passion was basketball, and he decided that he would feel more fulfilled as a basketball coach. He had always enjoyed the sport, and he found great delight inspiring young children. Once Dick rose above his programming, he no longer felt the need to make up for the person he was by lying or pretending to be something he was not.

Witnessing: A Path to Overcome

Compulsive Negativity

Leon wanted to be a musician, however, his negative mind told him that it was impossible, and he took a position at the Post Office. His destructive attitude caused difficulties early on the job, and in less than three months he was dismissed. Shortly after his release, his lover asked him to move out. Leon moved in with his mother, who became the primary target for venting his blame and negativity. Within two weeks of living alongside Leon's depression and verbal attacks, his mother had a stroke. When Leon went to visit her at the hospital, he upset her so much that she had a seizure, and he was asked not to return. In fear for her sister's well-being, Leon's aunt made an appointment for him to begin The Witnessing Technique, so that he could overcome his compulsive negativity.

When Leon called, he was invited to express how he was feeling. His first comment was, "Why, no one cares." Then he shut down, and the phone remained silent on his end for over ten minutes as he suffered through his own internal negativity. After some gentle coaxing, he finally shared that he felt misunderstood and emotionally unsupported. He was guided to close his eyes and allow his feelings to develop into an image, and the vision of a diabolical monster that sprayed acid from his mouth appeared. Leon enjoyed watching the monster as it maimed those he hated, which turned out to be anyone who crossed his path.

Leon was then asked why he hated everyone and he eventually shared that he felt insignificant in the midst of other people. He wanted to be a famous musician, but he did not believe that he ever would be. Leon was guided to allow his emotions to form into an image, and the vision of a terrified wolf that had been trapped and backed into a corner appeared. Every once in a while it would become courageous and snarl loudly, but then it would recede further into the corner and appear more distraught. *Leon's programming had no resolution for him. It simply prompted him to snarl and recede. He acted just like the wolf whenever he felt insignificant.*

Leon was guided to connect with the aspect of his consciousness that was able to observe the wolf. Once he had identified with his *Witnessing Self,* he felt immediately uplifted. For the first time in his life, Leon realized that he had the choice to rise above his pain and connect with an aspect of his consciousness that was eternally powerful and optimistic. This new experience felt promising to Leon, and he suggested that we apply the technique to work on his biggest problem—he did not know *who* he was or what purpose he had in life.

Leon was guided to allow the feeling of "not knowing who he was" to form into an image, and the vision of a ghost appeared. It hovered against a black background, lifeless and unexpressive. Once Leon had identified with his *Witnessing Self,* he shared that he felt omnipotent and substantial as the *witness,* but that his "ghost" felt weak and unsubstantial. The programming in his mind held only misery, but his *Witnessing Self* offered freedom and authority over his life.

When Leon realized that his *Witnessing Self* represented his **true self,** he was thrilled to finally have some sense of "self" with which to connect. He agreed to continue practicing the technique on his own. He was also encouraged to neutralize his thoughts each day. When he noticed negativity arising, he was guided to clap his hands or snap his fingers to shake himself out of it. The next step was to choose to be *neutral* about how he was feeling or thinking instead. Many times he had to shout NEUTRAL, aloud in order to remain centered, but the exercises worked and Leon found his mind becoming more peaceful each day. *Leon was not encouraged to move directly toward a positive thought, because such an action felt impossible to him and consequently made him angry. Those who suffer from compulsive* *negativity will experience much more success at rising above the mind by reaching for a neutral outlook on life before they try to move toward positive thoughts.*

As Leon continued practicing the technique, he experienced a profound increase in energy and many creative ideas began to flow through his imagination. He painted his mother's house for her and worked in her back field cultivating a thriving vegetable and flower garden. He also discovered that he had a talent for making flower pots in the shape of model airplanes. The neighbors liked his work so much that he was contracted to build some for them as well.

Within a few months of practicing the technique, Leon had reconnected with his creative energy in a profound way. This shift brought purpose and significance back into his life. As his confidence grew, he began playing his guitar and writing songs again, which eventually led to starting up a band. Once he was able to rise above his negative programming, he enjoyed every moment of life to its fullest.

Witnessing: A Path to Overcome

Compulsive Worry

Ian was an aspiring singer, songwriter in New York City. He was motivated, diligent, and aggressive. His two main goals in life were to become very successful with his career and to marry the perfect woman. Although he had received some positive comments about his work, no one was ready to represent him. After eight long years of persistently marketing himself, as well as singing in clubs and musical theater productions, he felt he was far from the success he craved. The same pattern presented itself in his love life. His girlfriends thought he tried very hard at being a good boyfriend, but he was not quite what they were looking for. The harder he tried, the more rejected and unimportant he felt. According to his mind, he just did not measure up.

From the moment Ian woke up, until the moment he fell asleep and even in his dreams, he would worry about his life and his career, fearing that he would die a lonely washed up "wanna be" in New York City and that no one would even notice he was gone. His mind was continually diminishing his chances of success.

One day Ian met up with an old acquaintance named Jerry at an audition. He noticed that Jerry's broken teeth had been repaired. He was wearing nice clothing for a change, and confidence exuded from his presence. Jerry shared that he had a high paying gig at a very ritzy club up town, and he had also signed with a record label that was about to release his first album. He looked and acted like a new person.

Ian was jealous and annoyed. He wanted the kind of success that Jerry had, but he felt hopeless that he would ever be able to reach his own goals. He asked Jerry how things turned around for him. Jerry said that his girlfriend had been practicing The Witnessing Technique for three years, and the shifts that occurred within her motivated him to practice *witnessing* himself. His luck began to change soon after he recognized his main program about struggle. As the *witness*, he had risen above it, and his life became much easier right away.

Ian was intrigued by what Jerry had to say, but he felt intimidated by the fact that his sessions would take place over the phone. He expressed worry about his phone bill, where he would find the time, and whether or not it would work for him. Jerry joked around and told Ian he should start working on his "worry program" right away.

When Ian called for his appointment, he was late. He made excuses by complaining about how hard his life was, emphasizing how worried he was there must be something wrong with him because he was not getting what he wanted. Ian was guided to close his eyes and allow his feelings to form into an image, and the vision of a marionette puppet appeared. With an angry tone, he described the puppet flailing around trying to get what it wanted, but someone else was holding his strings. Everyone who came in contact with the puppet had a chance to *string him along.* Ian became very frustrated. He said that it was about time someone *pulled some strings for him.* Even if he did his best, he believed he would always be a puppet in someone else's hands.

After Ian identified his programming and realized what it was doing to him, he became even more worried, jumping to the conclusion that he would never be able to change. Then he began a hostile diatribe, expressing that he worked very hard, and no one ever acknowledged how much he did or how good he was. He became increasingly angry as he spoke. Out of the blue he screamed into the phone, "I am doing the best I can do. I cannot try any harder or do any more." Ian was then asked what he thought he was being asked to try harder to do, and he replied that he felt he was being asked to do everything better, even The Witnessing Technique. His mind had interpreted that going further into the process without receiving a tremendous amount of praise first, meant that he had done something wrong. He was reassured that he had done everything correctly, and that he was making good progress. He broke into the sentence, however, berating himself, saying that he always screwed everything up.

Ian was guided to take a few deep breaths, and when he had finally calmed down, he allowed his worry to form into an image. The vision of a frantic girl appeared. She was pulling out her hair and pacing back and forth while she clenched her fists and muttered under her breath. She never solved anything and often made things much worse. Ian watched for over six minutes as the character expressed intense worry through her chaotic actions, and finally understood that it was his own behavior that held him back from success, not "those people" he expected to help him. When Ian had reached a neutral feeling about the frantic girl, he was guided to connect with the aspect of his consciousness that was able to observe the image, and he suddenly felt uncommonly carefree. Impressed by this drastic shift in energy, Ian agreed to practice the technique on his own throughout the week.

When Ian called for his next appointment, he shared that every time his mind jumped to the conclusion that his success was up to everyone who could pull strings for him, he recognized the marionette puppet programming and became the *witness* of it instead. He also realized how weak, pathetic, and "victim like" he became when the programming took a hold of him, and how repulsive this would be to a prospective employer. Once he understood that he could separate himself from the marionette programming and determine his own success, his new-found confidence made him much more appealing to audiences.

As Ian continued to work with the technique and *witness* his emotions, his self-esteem strengthened, and he stopped worrying about impressing every single person who could pull some strings and get him a job. Instead, he trusted his talent and invested more in his original voice and lyrics. For the first time in his career, he enjoyed himself. In the past he had been after the success of a singer, but as the *witness*, he was more interested in being true to himself and his original talent. Once he made that decision, his career took off, and his love life blossomed as well.

Witnessing: A Path to Overcome
The Compulsive Fear of Death

When Garth was first diagnosed with a terminal illness, he was put into a small hospice and given one month to live. Two years passed and he was still holding on. The nurses at the hospice determined that his pain had to be unbearable, but Garth refused to take any pain medication and his family did not know what to do. No one wanted him to go on suffering. The Lead Nurse had many conversations with him about dying, but he was too frightened to let go.

Garth's son arranged for his father to be taken through The Witnessing Technique at the hospice and he agreed as long as it did not coincide with, "I Love Lucy," his favorite show. Before the session began, Garth was telling funny stories, but once his audience was out of sight, he grasped on to the bedpost and let out a deep groan. The pain in his body could be seen clearly through his sallow gripping skin and the clenching expression on his ninety-six year old face. Garth opened his eyes briefly and winked, saying, "I can't hide this much longer." He gave a deep sigh and closed his eyes; preparing himself for the next half hour.

When he appeared more comfortable, Garth was gently invited to express his fears. His face took on a grim expression as his grip on the bedpost tightened, then he slowly shared that he could not bring himself to leave his body. He had almost succeeded a few times, but his fear kept pulling him back. He refused to take the pain medication because he wanted to choose when he was going to die. He did not wish to die _uncon-sciously_, filled with drugs. He wanted to watch and see what happened, calling it a "once in a lifetime chance viewing." Garth reasoned that if he could remain alert and awake when he left his body, he would have more control over where his spirit went, and he wanted to make sure it went to a nice place.

Garth was guided to allow his fear to take the form of an image, and the vision of a deep dark grave appeared. He could not see what was at the bottom, or if there was a bottom at all. There was a long silence and then Garth recalled his Sunday school teacher leading him into a dark cloakroom and whispering in his ear that he was a bad boy and he would go straight to hell, which she described as a deep dark pit of agony and eternal torture. Garth's eyes began to water as he looked out the window. He then shared that his whole life had changed that day. He never felt safe again. The fear of death occupied his mind from that moment forward.

In an attempt to assist Garth in rising above his pain, he was guided back inside to connect with his *Witnessing Self*. Garth was silent with closed eyes for quite a while—then shared that when he *identified* with *the observant* aspect of his being, (his *Witnessing Self*) he felt as though he had risen above the vision of the grave, as well as the old man lying in bed. "It does not look frightening at all from up here," Garth exclaimed, with a little chuckle. His face took on an expression of peace as he let go of his grip from the bedpost.

Garth was then asked which seemed more "real" to him: the experience of being the *Witness*, or the image of the grave? Garth chuckled to himself again, and then said that the only thing that felt real was his *Witnessing Self*, everything else appeared as though it were a dimming mirage.

Garth was becoming quite pale, so he was guided to allow his physical pain to form into an image, and the vision of a ripping torch appeared. It had a razor like fire blazing from one end and it ripped and jerked in the air. Once Garth was able to rise above the image, and identify with Pure Consciousness, his physical pain moved into the distance. He was still aware of it, but it was more numb and throbbing now, as apposed to hot and ripping. Garth had done enough for one afternoon, so he was asked to playfully practice connecting with his *Witnessing Self* for the next few days. He agreed and fell right to sleep.

Garth was bright and cheerful once again as he prepared for his second Witnessing session. He was feeling rather good physically and his spirits were high. When he was asked about his fear of death, Garth replied that he had been a fool his whole life to believe what some Sunday school teacher (who had no experience of the beyond herself,) had told him about death. Garth then shared that he felt carefree as long as he remained identified with his *Witnessing Self.* He admitted that he still did not know for certain what death was, but he had a growing suspicion that he had only been afraid of fear itself.

Garth had been having many dreams since his first Witnessing session, in which he experienced visions of light and freedom from his body. However, he still had fear that the old programming of the grave would grab at him at the last minute, and he wanted to feel completely confident before he was willing to consider leaving his body. Garth was once again led into the technique as he focused on his new fear, and the image of an old broken down machine appeared. The machine had many cylinders, bells and whistles on it, but Garth could not imagine what purpose it served, other than spinning a lot of wheels. The machine also seemed desperate to remain in control. It was tight and tense and attached to being in charge of what happened.

Garth was guided to identify with his *Witnessing Self,* and within a few minutes he began to laugh, sharing that the machine was his mind and that it was always spinning its wheels to appear useful, but that it really had no ability to provide Garth with what he needed when he died.

As he lay in bed identifying with his *Witnessing Self,* Garth described a feeling of grace sweeping over him. He felt weightless, free and excited about the beyond—certain that he was about to head off on an incredible journey with great adventures ahead. From this heightened perspective,

Garth was aware that he was neither the body nor the mind, but the aspect of his consciousness that could see his whole life. He felt confident that even if his body was to die, that his *Witnessing Self* would remain strong and the old machine spinning its wheels would not be able to interfere anymore. He had successfully identified with Pure Consciousness and risen above the fearful programming in his mind.

Garth left his body less than a week after his second session. His son shared that he had never seen his father look more peaceful. He died with a smile on his face. *By identifying with Pure Consciousness, we can die consciously and remain connected to the essence of our being which is eternal.*

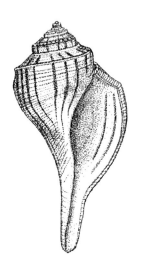

CHAPTER 8

Depression

Introduction

Suppressed emotions which build to the point of devastation, inhibiting an individual's ability to connect with or apply creative energy.

THE DEPRESSED PERSON IS LITERALLY PRESSED DOWN by their negative thoughts and emotions. Heavy clouds of untransformed experiences permeate their being and often lead to a severe lack of energy, an aversion to accomplish tasks, and in some cases no will to live at all.

The Witnessing Technique will support the depressed individual in rising above their repressed thoughts and emotions, as well as the mental programming which causes them to suppress or hold onto their feelings and thoughts in the first place. Physical activity, exciting goals, as well as the *intention* to be happy and filled with vitality, add further support for a rapid recovery.

Witnessing: A Path to Overcome

Depression Due to Hopelessness

Keira fell into a deep depression when her long term boyfriend Chuck suddenly decided he was going to marry her best friend Mary. When Keira received this information, she dropped out of college, quit her part time job, and stopped exercising and being social altogether. With each day that passed, Keira lost more of her will to live.

When Keira called for her appointment, her voice was a lifeless monotone. She had been taking sleeping pills for over five months. They had dulled her mind and created great difficulty for her to remain focused. After forty-five minutes of expressing her feelings, however, she finally connected with the rage she had been suppressing since the day Chuck left.

Keira was guided to allow her rage to form into an image, and the vision of a "cat woman" appeared. Her black head of hair stood out in rigid spikes as she hissed and clawed at Mary and Chuck before she ripped them to shreds. Keira watched her image vent her suppressed pain for over twelve minutes in her imagination; an experience that cleared her mind and relaxed her body. Impressed by the dramatic shift in her energy and clarity, Keira agreed to allow the image to express as much rage as possible throughout the week.

When Keira called for her next appointment, she was quite astonished to report that her rage had neutralized. She missed her anger, however, because it had made her feel more alive after almost nine months of feeling dead and depressed. Without the anger, her buried sadness had begun to surface. Keira was guided to allow her sadness to form into an image, and the vision of a lonely, abandoned water spring appeared. The spring was covered with a large rock, but it had found an opening and was now flowing with spring water tears that seemed to have no end. The symbolic release felt liberating to Keira, and she spent more time each day *witnessing* the spring until real tears began to flow from her own eyes. Along with her tears, a weightlessness arose within her lungs, as if a heavy boulder had been lifted away from her chest.

Once her anger and sadness had been neutralized, Keira found her most predominant emotion to be hopelessness. When she allowed her hopelessness to form into an image, the vision of an old, shriveled woman sitting in front of a decaying wedding cake with worms and mold covering it appeared in her mind. The vision reminded Keira of a *Dickens* character named *Miss Havisham.* She was wearing her wedding gown, which she had worn for the past fifty years since her groom stood her up on their wedding day. Her wedding dress had turned from white to a dusty gray, and the delicate lace had become coarse against her skin, leaving an unpleasant rash around her neck and wrists. Keira watched as the character sat brooding before the decaying cake, and suddenly she felt the ridiculousness of being a victim. As she allowed Miss Havisham to sit, mope, pout, and brood, Keira realized that according to her programming *she was doomed to be alone, unloved, unwanted and hopeless no matter what.*

"How could anyone love a martyr like that?" she exclaimed. "No wonder Chuck left me. Mary would never be such a victim. She would have moved on to the next great guy as quickly—"

Keira stopped mid sentence and was silent for a moment. When she began to speak again, she shared that she was shocked by how easily she was able to talk about Chuck and Mary. She could see the whole situation from a higher perspective at that moment, and she understood why Chuck had left her for someone who was always delightful to be around. The awareness of her own part in the break-up made Keira less resentful toward Chuck and Mary. Instead of getting down on herself, she felt inspired to change.

Keira was guided to connect with the aspect of her consciousness that was able to observe the image of Miss Havisham, and within a few moments she was bubbling over with enthusiasm, expressing how riveting and freeing her *Witnessing Self* felt. As the *witness*, she was excited about life again.

Keira's recovery was very speedy after her first view of Miss Havisham. The next day she was out exercising, calling old friends, looking into getting back into college, and finding a job. Without the mental programming that she would always be unloved and unwanted, Keira reconnected with her true power and took charge of her life. Any time she finds her mind shifting into victim mode, she *witnesses* the Miss Havisham character and quickly gets back on track by identifying with Pure Consciousness, which always makes her feel strong and overflowing with love.

Witnessing: A Path to Overcome Depression due to Self-Loathing

In his teens, Sanders began fantasizing about holding hands and being seen with famous movie stars. In his visions, crowds would roar with approval at Sanders, and he would feel better for a short while. Once out of his daydream, however, he found himself more disillusioned with his real life.

He had subscriptions to many tabloid magazines and lived vicariously through their gossip. One day he discovered that the celebrity of his dreams had recently married. To escape his pain, Sanders ate boxes of chocolates and watched sad love movies every night while his parents tried to sleep in the next room. Sometimes he would stay up weeping until four or five in the morning and would be unable to make it to school the next day.

In desperation, he wrote love letters to the celebrity with whom he was obsessed. He delivered them along with bouquets of flowers, chocolates, and balloons almost every week for six months with no reply. Depressed over the lack of response, Sanders became despondent and was unable to get out of bed. He rarely made it to class, so he finally decided to drop out of school. One of his teachers encouraged him to continue and suggested The Witnessing Technique as a support system for his despair.

When Sanders called, he shared that his depression was rooted in trying very hard to get what he wanted without receiving anything for his efforts. He closed his eyes and allowed his feelings to form into an image, and the vision of a huge boulder covered in tar and nails formed in his mind. In an exasperated tone, he described the boulder as burdensome, irritating, and unworthy. Every time it moved forward toward its goal, it would immediately roll backwards again and lose any progress it had made.

Sanders was asked to watch the boulder until he felt neutral, which took quite a while, because he was very attached to hating it. *The boulder represented a program in his mind which made him believe that he could never get what he wanted, because he was worthless.* Astounded by the subtle symbolism in his psyche, Sanders agreed to *witness* the image all week in order to distance himself from its effects.

When Sanders called for his next appointment, his predominant emotion was anger, so he was guided to allow his anger to form into an image. The vision of *Gollum* from *Lord of the Rings* appeared. The Gollum character had flames spewing out from his eyes, mouth, and fingers. He wanted to rip apart everyone who did not applaud him or give him a chance to prove how special he was. Sanders watched the character and expressed that it was ugly, worthless, and unwanted. It had no hope of ever being loved. When he stepped into the *witnessing* position, however, he felt at peace, and it became clear to him that he was wasting his life as he waited for others to make him feel better about himself.

Within a few days of this breakthrough, he started waking up early and going for morning walks, instead of sleeping until noon and eating chocolates all day to escape his depression. Before he went to sleep each night, he would review the day and look for any programming that he could recognize. Then he would *witness* the images before he fell asleep. Consequently, he would wake up feeling much more in control of his life.

When a strong emotion arose for Sanders during the day, he would immediately allow the emotion to form into an image and observe the symbolism. Then he would identify with his *Witnessing Self* and detach completely from the programming.

These small internal shifts transformed his life. Within seven weeks of practicing the technique, he not only perceived his life as an opportunity to create whatever he wanted, but he also felt lovable and important simply because he was alive. He did not need the attention of a celebrity or the applause from a crowd. He was no longer identified with the self-loathing and worthlessness his programming had projected on him.

CHAPTER 9

Eating Disorders

Introduction

A determined disconnection from the natural rhythm
and flow of the bodies nutritional and biological needs.

WE ARE BORN WITH A REVERENCE FOR OUR OWN BODY and a deep connection to what it needs. When a baby is hungry, it will cry for food. When a baby is satisfied, it will refuse to eat. Our bond with the body is part of our intrinsic nature before the ego intervenes.

We have unnatural desires because we have mental programming. They are one and the same. People turn into food addicts, anorexics, bulimics, or compulsive eaters when the mind decides to find comfort or control through the misuse of the body.

Perfect health and perfect weight are our natural inheritance. By rising above the distorted programming in the mind and identifying with Pure

Consciousness, we can realign with our original state of grace and live free from any preoccupation with food and diet.

Witnessing: A Path to Overcome

Anorexia

Sheila was a very active sophomore involved with school clubs and athletics. She was attractive, intelligent, and popular. When she joined the cheerleading team, she was chosen as the acrobat—to be tossed in the air and held up by the rest of the squad throughout the routines. Consequently, she devoted most of her time attending ballet and gymnastics lessons in order to be the best she could be.

During exams, however, Sheila was not as active as usual. She became anxious while studying, and calmed herself with hot cocoa and brownies. After a week of cramming, Sheila showed up to cheerleading practice and noticed that her gym shorts were a bit tight. When the squad did their regular routine of throwing her in the air, one student complained that Sheila was too heavy and suggested they choose another girl who was lighter for her position. Although this was mentioned as a joke, Sheila took it to heart and became obsessed with the thought of being as light and thin as possible, so she cut her caloric intake down to 400 calories per day.

Within one week her gym shorts were loose again, and the cheerleading squad mentioned how light she was during practice. Sheila was thrilled and felt encouraged to become even lighter, so she began eating even less. She substituted her daily apple with broth and did three hundred sit ups each night. She lost twelve pounds in seven weeks and received a lot more attention from boys, as well as many compliments at her cheerleading practices and ballet lessons.

After rehearsal one day, the boy Sheila had a crush on, Colin, asked her out. She could not believe her luck. Once she started dating him, however, she discovered that he was very controlling with her time. She dropped out of gymnastics classes in order to meet his demands. To make certain that she would not put on weight, she took up running morning and night.

Colin invited her out for Root Beer floats every day at lunch. She did not want to drink them, but he stated that he hoped she was not one of those boring girls that refused to enjoy fun food with him. Sheila felt pressured and decided she would drink the floats and work out twice as hard each night.

As Sheila spent more time with Colin, she noticed that he would often tease anyone who was not quite thin enough for his standards. He also made a habit of telling her that she was almost perfect, just ten pounds to go and she would be his dream girl. Sheila felt fat and hideous every time Colin mentioned her weight, and she wanted more than anything to be ten pounds lighter. At this point, she had already lost sixteen pounds, but every time she looked in the mirror, she would agonize over the parts of her body that held any fat, and she'd punch them. She began taking an over-the-counter drug that was marketed to help people lose weight by suppressing their appetite and speeding up their metabolism. After taking it for ten days, she experienced dizzy spells, but she refused to stop taking the drug, because she feared that she might gain weight.

One day during cheerleading practice Sheila fainted, and the paramedics were called. Her heart had irregular palpitations, and she was very anemic. She was taken to the hospital for closer examination. After a thorough check up, her doctor asked her how long she had been anorexic. Sheila was shocked. In her mind she was still chubby, and this man thought she was anorexic? She became angry and shot back that he was crazy. When the doctor put Sheila on the scale, she weighed in at 101 pounds, and she was

5 foot 4. The doctor then asked her if she was taking any weight-loss drugs. Sheila felt embarrassed, so she lied and said no. Her doctor, however, still warned against the damage they could cause and shared that he was very concerned about her health and her heart. He also encouraged her to get some help with her emotions.

The next week Sheila met up with Colin at the ice crème parlor. He seemed distant and did not pay much attention to her. His friends were there, and they were making jokes about a girl named Julie. They chided Colin for turning red when everyone saw him talking to her after school the day Sheila had been taken to the hospital. Colin avoided Sheila's glance, but she understood that he had found another girl.

Sheila was devastated. She was certain Colin did not like her anymore because she was too fat, so she refused to eat for the next three days. She went for a run on the third night and passed out in a field. Her parents found her at one o'clock in the morning. She was freezing and hardly breathing. Once again she was taken to the hospital. The doctor recommended she begin working with The Witnessing Technique, and her mother made an appointment for her right away.

When Sheila arrived, she sat down with her hands tightly folded, and then she looked up with terror in her eyes. "You are not going to make me start eating are you?" was her first question. The panic in her voice was horrific. She was terrified of putting on weight and appeared to feel totally out of control.

When Sheila was asked to express her most intense feeling, she closed her eyes and tears rolled down her cheeks. Her most intense feeling was heartbreak. She was guided to allow her emotion to form into an image, and the vision of a body that had a big hole in it appeared in her mind. The heart and stomach were missing, as if they had been shot out by a big canon. The body had no defense against the outside forces and no strength to move forward far enough to reach something it wanted. When asked what the body was reaching for, Sheila answered, "Love." She went on to say that the body was empty and ready to die.

Sheila opened her eyes and shared that she feared she would never be loved, because her body was not perfect, and she was petrified of gaining weight. She was guided to close her eyes and allow her fear to form into an image. After a few moments a big glob appeared. It was gooey and round and "glumpy" in Sheila's words. The glob looked like a big fat particle. It turned red in shame and tried to hide, but it was too big and glumpy to avoid being seen.

Sheila was disgusted with the image, so she was directed to observe it until she felt neutral. Once this had been accomplished, she was guided to identify with the aspect of her consciousness that was able to observe the glob, and she realized right away that the image was only a mental projection based on her self-hatred. As the *witness*, she felt more kindness toward her body, and she immediately wanted to care for herself in a more loving manner.

With this new found confidence, Sheila opened up about some difficulty she was having at home. When she was forced to have dinner with her family, she was unable to remain detached from how ugly and hated her father made her feel. Sheila was guided to allow these feelings to form into an image, and the vision of a girl wrapped up in bandages like a Mummy appeared. The image felt unable to express itself, and it wanted to escape from everything. Sheila was guided to connect with her *Witnessing Self* and experience her true power as she observed the helpless Mummy, and she immediately gave a sigh of relief. She had never considered that she was allowed to detach from the pain. She thought her father wanted her to feel frightened and hurt, and she did not want to disappoint him.

As the *witness*, Sheila was able to feel compassion for her father for being so angry all the time. She also recognized that she was not responsible for his anger, and she was not the ugly, fat image she thought her father portrayed her to be. Once she started observing her ego's pain instead of identifying with it, she was able to remain confident in her father's presence by maintaining her connection with Pure Consciousness.

Sheila continued to *witness* her programming every time she experienced her fear of getting fat. Within two months she had reached a very healthy and slender weight for her body, and she looked fantastic. She felt slim, strong, and beautiful for the first time in her life, and she no longer experienced any fear of getting fat or of being ugly. She finally felt safe with food.

As Sheila progressed with The Witnessing Technique, her perspective on her relationship with Colin completely changed. Colin had treated her as brutally as her father had, and it felt familiar. Her attraction to him was based on her self-destructive programming. Deep down, she believed that if she could be loved by someone as controlling and judgmental as Colin, their relationship would take away the pain of her controlling, judgmental father not loving her. However, Colin simply ingrained a deeper sense of self-hatred in Sheila, and her heartache had grown more intense.

Once the old programming no longer had any power over her, Sheila was able to rely on her opinion of herself instead of the opinion of others who mistreated her. She rose above her struggle with anorexia and self-hatred, and she remains a strong, healthy athlete to this day.

Witnessing: A Path to Overcome

Bulimia

When Kate was signed on as a primary dancer with a large ballet company, she was partnered with one of the smaller men, because she was very tiny. In her second year, however, she had a four-inch growth spurt. She was happy about it, but her dance partner was not. He mentioned that she had put on weight, and he was having difficulty balancing her. Kate was horrified. She wanted to keep her position within the company, which in her mind meant that she had to dance just as gracefully with her partner as she had for the previous two years.

She began scrutinizing everything she ate. When she denied herself certain foods, her mind would obsess over consuming that specific food, and within a few days she would binge on everything from which she had abstained. She was putting on weight instead of losing it, and she became more frantic with each passing day. Unfortunately, the only thing that seemed to calm her nerves was eating.

A big performance was coming up in which Kate would be a featured dancer, and she wanted it to be perfect. Her parents were flying in to watch, and she became even more obsessed with her weight and appearance. She decided to fast on lemon juice and water for three days before the show with just a small piece of fish for lunch the day of the performance.

The show went well, and Kate's performance was somehow spectacular, but after the show she was ravenous. She went out for dinner with her parents and used her will power to eat only a small portion. She even refused the chocolate cake for dessert. In the morning, however, all Kate could think about was chocolate cake. She had two days off, and she convinced herself that it would be all right to have a treat after she had worked so hard all weekend. She purchased an entire chocolate cake and ate the whole thing. Afterwards, she worried about what her partner would do if she had put on weight over their break, so she ran to the bathroom and made herself throw up. The next day Kate stepped on the scale and discovered that she had *not* gained one pound. She was delighted and thought to herself that eating and purging was a good trick to keep her happy with what she wanted to eat, and still remain trim.

Over the next week rehearsals went well, and Kate employed her bingeing and purging technique four days in a row. By the weekend, she felt exhausted and was unable to get out of bed. When Monday's rehearsal rolled around, she was unable to keep up with the music, and her body was not dancing with its usual gracefulness and vitality. This behavior pattern continued for six months. Her health and energy slowly deteriorated, and she was replaced with another feature dancer for the fall shows.

Kate was devastated. She took a leave of absence from the company and went home to visit her family. She felt trapped and suffocated at home. The worse she felt, the more she wanted something sweet, and a lot of it. One weekend her parents went out of town, and Kate planned two days of bingeing and purging. Before her parents left, she fasted on water and lemon juice for three days to prepare herself for bingeing without guilt. The moment her parents were out the door, Kate ran up to her room and started in on the treats she had been thinking about for three days. She ate so much so fast that her body was unable to process the food, and her spleen almost ruptured. Kate was taken to the hospital in an ambulance, and her parents were called back home.

When her parents entered her bedroom, they found the empty wrappers and unfinished cakes and cookies she had planned on devouring over the weekend. Kate's doctor suggested that she had an eating disorder called bulimia, but Kate assured everyone that she was just depressed, and that everything would be different now, because she had learned her lesson. Nonetheless, her father was adamant that she receive professional help, and he sent her in for a Witnessing session.

When Kate arrived, she sat down very gracefully and pulled a pillow up to cover her body. She was embarrassed to admit why she was at the session, but offered that she really wanted to be healthy, and she wanted to get her cravings for sugar out of her mind. Kate was asked to recall what emotion took hold of her each time before she binged, and she shared that it was panic. She was guided to allow the emotion to form into an image, and a panicking figure zooming around in all directions, screaming, and shoveling food into her mouth appeared. The image was petrified. Everything seemed to "freak her out," in Kate's words. Kate was guided to identify with the aspect of her consciousness that was able to observe the panicking character. Once she had established a connection with her *Witnessing Self*, she recognized that her mind's only solution to escape her panic was soothing food.

The image of the panic-stricken girl made it clear to Kate that deep down she felt terrified, inconsolable, and unsafe in life. When she identified with her *Witnessing Self*, however, she felt calm, centered, and peaceful. Kate agreed to watch the image and disconnect from the panic as much as possible every time she felt her urge to binge. She also agreed to seek out the help of a nutritionist or a doctor who could assist her in regulating her sugar cravings by balancing the blood sugar levels in her body.

When Kate arrived for her next session, she reported that she had been able to observe herself mentally turning into the dramatic image and freaking out about what to do, but she was unable to change her behavior. Kate's body was so out of balance from her sugar bingeing and purging, that she experienced cravings and physical reactions similar to those of a diabetic. She felt as though she might pass out, or freak out, if she could not get sugar into her body fast enough. This had to be addressed in order for her to proceed with her healing.

The Witnessing Technique will raise awareness and offer a magnificent alternative to falling into the emotional rut of any destructive programming. To support this process, the body and its imbalances must be addressed as well. Kate had extremely low levels of blood sugar, which added a biological aspect to her cravings. What had begun as programming in her mind had manifested itself as a physical health concern.

Kate eventually found the courage to work with a nutritionist who was versed in helping people with eating disorders and blood sugar imbalances by employing Applied Kinesiology, a technique which accesses the true response the body has to an outside stimulus. Instead of allowing her mind to decide what was appropriate for her healing, she was muscle tested in order to determine what foods her body tested positively to. She was put on a diet which consisted mostly of lean protein, bitter vegetables, and olive oil. She was instructed to eat a small meal every two hours and comfortably drink as much water as she could each day. Kate also started seeing an acupuncturist, and she received a massage once a week to help calm her nerves.

Once Kate's physical health had improved and her blood sugar levels had stabilized, she reported that her body no longer experienced desperate sugar cravings. When she felt nervous, however, she did not know how to calm herself down without eating something, even if it was just a little bit. She was guided to allow her anxiety to form into an image in her mind, and once again her panicking figure appeared. When she was guided to identify with her *Witnessing Self,* she immediately felt calm and centered. She was then asked if her tranquil experience as the *witness,* could take the place of food when she was anxious. Kate looked very surprised, and then she answered, "Yes!" She sat quietly for a few minutes, and then she let out a sigh of relief and said, "I get it now. All I have to do is align with the real me, the *witness*, and the programming cannot affect me anymore." Kate was right.

When Kate arrived for her next session, she shared that as long as she remained the *witness* of her anxiety, she was able to walk away from unnecessary eating by sitting down in a quiet space and observing her anxiety instead. As she watched the panicking character in her mind, she allowed it to express and vent her fears for her. Afterwards she felt peaceful, healthy, and proud of herself for rising above the craziness of her mental programming. By the time her character had vented her anxiety, Kate's desire to shovel food into her mouth in order to feel in control of her anxiety had passed.

As the *witness*, Kate was attracted to new foods that she had never found interesting before. They gave her high quality energy with very few calories. The profound wisdom of her *Witnessing Self* was naturally guiding her toward healthier choices. Kate joined with a new dance company and discovered that her confidence and stability as a dancer had also increased. Once she learned to identify with the peaceful grace of Pure Consciousness, her entire life transformed.

Witnessing: A Path to Overcome Compulsive Eating Patterns

Jane was quiet and private by nature and subservient around others. She also became nervous when she mingled with the crowds at her college. Consequently, she would self-medicate her anxiety with food. Even when she was stuffed full from dinner, she would put a whole quart of pudding by her study books and dip into it every few minutes. The impulses in Jane's mind made it impossible for her to stop eating, even when she felt her stomach might burst.

After her first year of college, Jane became very self-conscious, because she had put on so much weight. The only clothes that fit her were loose sweat pants and baggy shirts, so she stopped putting on makeup or doing her hair in an attempt to blend into the background. The worse she felt about herself, the more her mind would focus on food. Even while she was in class, her mind would become agitated without something to chew on. The compulsive thought of food had control over her life.

Jane embarked upon one diet after another, trying to curb her obsession with food, but nothing worked. She continued to put on at least three pounds each month. Jane's roommate, Karen, was thin and fit and never seemed to desire food unless she was hungry. Even then, she would only take a small amount and leave most of it uneaten on her plate.

In desperation, Jane asked her roommate how she was able to move through life without any attachment to food. Karen told her about The Witnessing Technique. She admitted that she had suffered from an obsession with sugar only five years earlier, so Jane made an appointment right away.

When Jane arrived for her first session, she was disheveled and shy. She hid her face behind long bangs and rarely looked up. She seemed happy to be able to close her eyes throughout most of the exercises and spoke very little. When she was asked about her emotions, she expressed a strong feeling of nervousness. As she sat with the nervousness, she felt afraid of being in her body. In fact, it felt dangerous just being alive. Jane was guided to allow her feelings to form into an image, and a figure that appeared to be a hologram appeared. When she observed the image, it became nervous and turned more solid. As it became solid, it became frantic to disappear. Her character did not feel comfortable having a body. It was big, clumsy, and afraid to be seen.

Jane observed the character for quite a while and watched as it tried to disappear, or in her words, "stop existing." The character was very concerned with staying out of the way of others. When the image became aware of another presence, it dropped its head, certain to be judged. This image brought up intense emotions for Jane, and she spent the rest of her session exploring what the image represented symbolically. This helped her release more of her nervous tension.

Jane practiced the technique all week, and by the sixth day of *witnessing* her hologram character, she was able to observe her image without emotional attachment. Once she felt no emotion about the image, her desire for food diminished tremendously. *Compulsive eating had been a way of avoiding what she did not want to see within herself.* Once she had faced a core fear, her programming had less control over her.

When Jane arrived for her next session, she had her hair pulled back from her face, and she was wearing a beautiful dress. She appeared calm and happy, and she sat down eager to look inside once again. The emotion that had been coming up for her recently had been the fear of her own power. When she closed her eyes and allowed her fear to form into an image, a vastness appeared. It was dark with twinkling stars, similar to the cosmos, and she felt lost in it.

Jane was invited to watch the image until she felt neutral. Then she was guided to connect with the aspect of her consciousness that was able to observe the image. Once she had identified with her *Witnessing Self,* she shared that the original vastness of the image felt daunting, because it was an outside source of energy that felt more powerful than she was. As the *witness,* however, she sensed that she could never be overpowered or controlled by anything. She was a part of everything, yet conscious of her own unique vibration.

Her new profound connection with Pure Consciousness strengthened her self-esteem, and her nervousness was quickly replaced by a sense of deep inner peace. Her fear of being overpowered, *which was the emotion that had instigated her compulsive eating*, no longer troubled her. Within three weeks of practicing The Witnessing Technique diligently, she found that the only time she ever considered eating was when she was hungry, which was a huge breakthrough for her, since she could not recall ever experiencing balance and connection with her body in her life. She also felt a desire to interact more openly with others, and over the course of eight months she released all the weight she had put on during her two years at college. As the *witness*, she saw herself from a higher perspective, and began to live as a new person. She was happy, light, confident, and carefree.

Witnessing: A Path to Overcome Food Addiction

Rachel had been heavy most of her life. As a small child, family members poked fun at her plumpness. School mates gave her chubby nick names, and cruel acquaintances pointed out the fact that she was overweight regularly.

Through the years she undertook lengthy fasts and received colonics and fancy cellulite removal techniques. Often she would work out for four to five hours a day and then collapse in desperation and eat everything she wanted for weeks on end. These extremes turned into bulimia and anorexia, and Rachel found herself losing and gaining fifty to sixty pounds a year.

In her thirties, she experienced digestive difficulties and decided to stop the extreme behavior. Consequently, she began eating on the Zone Diet. Every time she reached a relatively normal weight, however, her cravings would become unexplainably ravenous, and she would find herself eating two Zone meals every three hours instead of one. If someone commented on how slender she looked, Rachel would immediately run home and eat to the point of bursting. If the scale showed she had lost a few pounds, she would crave the most fattening foods possible and gobble them down. No matter how much effort Rachel put into losing weight, her mental programming would always force her to gain it back.

Rachel tried hypnotherapy, surgery, psychotherapy, and counseling, but she had the same results. Each time she reached a good weight, she would gain it all back more quickly than she had lost it. Eventually she decided to experiment with The Witnessing Technique to discover what programming caused her relapses.

When Rachel called for her appointment, she was asked to remember those times when she had become slender, so that she could locate the determining emotion that had inspired her to eat her way back to a heavy weight. She found it difficult to describe what the feeling was. The closest she could come was to say that when she looked in the mirror and saw her slender self, she felt sick to her stomach. She was revolted and disgusted.

Rachel was guided to close her eyes and allow her feelings to form into an image, and the vision of a frumpy girl appeared. She had her head bent low to the ground, and she was ashamed of the way she looked. When Rachel was guided to connect with the aspect of her consciousness that was able to observe the image, she found the shift from identifying with the image to identifying with her *Witnessing Self* to be quite a welcome relief.

As a detached observer, Rachel was invited to discern what the image symbolized in her mind. The programming was very simple. Rachel believed that she was fat. Her mind remained constant with this *vision of self.* Whenever a different vision appeared, such as a thin Rachel, her programming made her feel extremely uncomfortable, as if she was no longer herself, but in someone else's body; a prospect that revolted her. She had to eat ravenously to gain weight as quickly as possible to match up again with her fat self-image.

Once Rachel was able to *witness* her programming, it no longer had any power over her. This freedom often made her laugh aloud, because it was so easy. The big powerful monster to which she had always succumbed in the past, was meek and helpless in the wake of her strong *Witnessing Self*. She enjoyed having power over the programming which had tortured her for most of her life.

Rachel was amazed by how easily her desire for fattening foods disappeared. She realized first hand that the mind forms cravings based on how we see ourselves. *The individual with a fat self-image will crave different foods than a person with a slender self-image. The body simply represents a blueprint of our psyche.* Once she had risen above her fat self-image, she felt that her taste buds had been replaced with someone else's. All she wanted was healthy food that offered energy and weight loss.

Within five months, Rachel had reached a very healthy weight, and this time she experienced no cravings whatsoever when she fit into her size-six dresses. Even when people noticed how slender she was, she felt no desire to eat. As of this publishing, it has been eight years since Rachel reached her size-six body, and she remains slender and healthy to this day.

Witnessing: A Path to Overcome *Self-Destructive Eating*

Self-love is the root of all beauty and balance. When we condemn or attempt to battle an aspect of the body, we are moving in the opposite direction of self-love. Instead of determining to fight the body, we must overcome the programming which causes self-hatred in the first place. Once that is alleviated, a beautiful body will follow.

Janet had been dieting and yo-yoing for most of her life. She had gained and lost more than 110 pounds in the previous year alone. Before she was introduced to The Witnessing Technique, Janet was certain that she had just been born fat and there was no hope of ever having the body that she really wanted. Every time she looked at her reflection, she threw hatred darts at her physique through the mirror, wishing she could rip the fat off and burn it. She loathed her body and begrudged it every chance she had.

On the verge of another self-destructive binge, Janet came in for an emergency session. It was very difficult to begin the technique, however, because her ego was using its tricks to break Janet's desire to change. She was frantic, weepy, petrified, hostile, blameful, and incredulously needy. (All are typical signs of ego control.) Her programming counted on her to fall back and let it take over again.

When Janet was finally able to close her eyes and move inside, she allowed the desperate feelings of destructive desire to form into an image. The vision of an hysterical blubber-woman appeared. The woman was "ugly and unlovable," in Janet's words. She was then guided to connect with the aspect of her consciousness that was able to observe the character. Once she had identified with her *Witnessing Self*, she felt more at ease, because she knew that the image was only a symbolic representation of how she saw herself according to her programming. This idea of self made her want to punish her body for being so unlovable, ugly, and fat.

As long as Janet wanted to punish herself, her programming would force her to eat the most fattening foods she could find as the worst form of self-punishment possible. In the past, she would force down a bag of cookies that she did not enjoy one bit, in a furious act of self-hatred that compelled her to eat every last morsel with self-disgust and self-hatred every bite along the way.

As soon as she moved into the *witnessing* position, the opposing forces of the ego, which urged her toward self-sabotage, dropped. She was shocked. Her desperate urge to eat destructively had completely evaporated, and she suddenly felt peaceful and fulfilled inside.

Janet had called the ego's bluff, and instead of backing off and giving it back its old control, she'd faced it with everything she had. From that point forward, whenever she found she was on the verge of self-sabotage, she would sit down and watch the blubber image try to self-destruct and take her with it. Each time she applied the technique, her *Witnessing Self* proved to be far more powerful than the programming that had destroyed her chances of success in the past.

As Janet became more familiar with her *Witnessing Self*, she understood that loving herself and treating herself with reverence and compassion were superior transformation techniques. Her previous bully approach, had only caused her more self-loathing.

Janet continued to shed an average of four pounds per month for one year. She was surprised that it was not difficult to do physically. For the first time in her life, she reached her ideal weight, and she maintains it easily to this day. *No matter how far away you have gone from your true perfection, The Witnessing Technique will guide you toward your most beautiful self.*

CHAPTER 10

Obsession

Romantic Obsession

*The projection of an image onto another person
with the expectation they will fulfill a fantasy.*

THE ROMANTICALLY OBSESSED INDIVIDUAL lives with an intense longing to possess a specific person of their choosing. They believe they are pursuing love itself, when in fact they are pursuing an idea in their psyche. They have already put a face to love, instead of allowing love to show its face.

The mind of the obsessed must view their chosen one as an object to be attained, versus the real person they are, in order to continue enjoying their fantasy. Imagination feeds their passion and fascination. Once the object of their infatuation becomes real, with their human qualities shining through, the obsessed will feel let down. When faced with rejection, the obsessive mind may become frantic. Their hope for wholeness has once again been lost, and what they had mistaken as love may quickly turn to hate.

Root of Attraction

Those with an obsessive mind will be drawn to the very people who will ignite their core fears, which is how the programming in the mind orchestrates our longing. People programmed to believe they are unwanted and unworthy of love, will become obsessed with someone who is unable to love or want them. Individuals who are programmed to believe they are bad will become obsessed with someone who finds only fault in them. The person programmed to fear deprivation may choose the perfect individual to deprive them of love and attention. A healthy mutually loving relationship will only occur between individuals who have risen above their programming.

Jilted Obsession

Many people become obsessed with a partner they once dated. If the relationship ended without the closure one individual needed, an obsession to reclaim and prove themselves to the other may exist. The obsessed will strive to better themselves by becoming more appealing, attractive, powerful, accomplished, or famous in order to woo their lost love back into their web.

Primal Obsession

In the case of Primal Obsession, people become infatuated with those who subconsciously represent the image of their mother or father or both. This sort of Obsession can be the most dangerous, because they are convinced the person they desire is their "soul mate." Yet, it is only the unhealed part of them which yearns for the emotional fulfillment of being loved by someone who represents their programmed idea of intimacy from childhood—even if this programming is based in an abusive familiarity.

Service Obsession

The fear of being alone often creates a desire to find someone to cling to. The Service Obsessed are afraid to live for themselves and instead choose to live for another. Their devotion is a barter in which they relinquish responsibility for loving themselves and leave it up to others. This barter can never fulfill the deep emptiness which arises from abandoning oneself. As a result, disappointment and resentment plague their lives.

Social Climber Obsession

Social Climbers want to exploit others in order to fulfill their own inadequacies. These people become obsessed with someone who they view as out of their league; often a movie star, prominent figure, or someone very wealthy, powerful, or outrageously attractive. Intensely driven by insecurity, they will do anything to acquire their prize, and they often become bored with their "beloved" once a greater prize appears on the horizon.

Unrequited Obsession

Obsession can arise due to the fear of being in an intimate relationship. Fantasizing about the perfect person who is unattainable is safe. The lust and pleasure of attraction are experienced, yet no opportunity exists for real rejection or intimacy. It is a fantasy which can go on indefinitely; therefore it is comfortable and predictable.

Witnessing: A Path to Overcome

Jilted Obsession

Serena met John at a restaurant they both frequented. At first she was not very interested in him, but he pursued her aggressively until she agreed to have dinner with him. After two weeks of dating, Serena felt certain that John was the man for her, but he expressed interest in remaining single and dating other women. From this moment forward, Serena was obsessed with regaining the feeling of having John want her as badly as he had in the beginning.

Intent on knowing all there was to know about him, she began secretly stalking him. Every once in a while she would follow him into a restaurant, then pretend to bump into him just so she could look into his eyes. John was always pleasant, but he never asked her out again.

Serena went on in this manner for fifteen years. During that time John married and started a family, but she held on to the belief that he could not possibly love his wife as much as he had loved her. After the birth of his fourth child, however, Serena started wondering how long she would have to wait before he realized he had chosen the wrong woman. One day Serena saw John out with his family, and he looked very happy. She began to contemplate suicide, but then she realized that she did not want to die. She wanted John or his wife to die.

Serena came in for an appointment at her most hopeless point. Sobbing hysterically, she shared that her deepest pain was rooted in the feeling of *not being chosen*, which had made her feel *unwanted* and *unloved*. She was guided to allow her pain to form into an image, and a gloomy figure hunched over in the corner of a dark room appeared. The figure was brooding and depressed. It was neither male nor female, nor did it have a face. It was a nondescript, pathetic energy that was certain love would never enter its experience, so it remained depressed and dismal in the corner, bearing its eternal pain. *According to her programming, nothing was going to change, so she was certain to die alone and unloved.*

Serena was guided to connect with the aspect of her consciousness that was able to observe the image. Once she had identified with her *Witnessing Self,* she felt free and light in comparison to the character of doom her mind had been projecting. As the *witness,* Serena also felt worthy and lovable, no longer desperate for someone else to validate her.

Eager to maintain her new feelings of self-worth, Serena practiced The Witnessing Technique every time she felt herself move into the longing she had for John. Eventually, the gloomy, hopeless character lost its grip over her. Within a few days she felt freer, lighter, happier, and more excited about life. By the end of the week, she was ready to start walking in the park again. She also became involved with social events and opened up to meeting new people.

Once her programming no longer had control over her fate, available men began pursuing her, and for the first time in her life, she felt lovable enough to choose a man who would be good for her, as opposed to becoming attached to the first man who showed some interest.

Witnessing: A Path to Overcome

Primal Obsession

Chloe was a published author of numerous cook books and a chef at her own five-star restaurant. When she turned thirty-three, she became obsessed with Brian, a young man she met at a party. He showed no interest in her, but she was certain they were soul mates, because she had such intense feelings toward him.

Chloe received Brian's e-mail address from a friend and sent a message asking him out on a date. He did not remember Chloe from the party, so he responded by telling her that he was in a relationship and had no interest in dating anyone else. Undaunted, Chloe instructed her assistant to gather the telephone numbers and addresses for Brian and his family members, so that she could invite them to her next big party.

She spent months planning a huge celebration to impress Brian and give herself the opportunity to spend time with him. On the hopeful night of the event, however, Brian was a no-show. Chloe was able to mingle with a few of Brian's family members, and she formed a connection by offering them invitations to important events where they would be treated as V.I.P.'s. Brian's family felt honored by Chloe's generosity and became friendly with her. This connection gave Chloe access to information about Brian on a regular basis, and she made a point of showing up uninvited to all his events. Once his family realized Chloe was stalking Brian, they stopped giving out his personal information. In desperation, Chloe embarked upon *Brian Rituals*. These were ceremonies to invoke the angels to help Brian realize how much he loved her. She never once considered that Brian was sincerely uninterested in her.

Every coincidence or symbolic image that reminded her of Brian was perceived as a sign from God that she was getting closer to being with him. If she had a customer who complimented the chef and his name was

Brian, Chloe believed that the Universe was telling her Brian really loved her. If she turned on the radio and there was a song that reminded her of Brian, she believed that it was a sign he was thinking of her. If she passed by a billboard or a movie theater and the name Brian was displayed, she thought that Existence wanted her to be reassured Brian would always be in her life.

This is common behavior for an obsessive ego. The mind becomes so focused on its desires that it will attract information and circumstances that symbolize the obsession. These coincidental reminders of Brian were not signs that Brian loved Chloe, as she had happily assumed. They were signs that her mind was compulsively thinking about him, desperately seeking information to support her obsessive theory that they would eventually be together.

After months of badgering, Brian finally agreed to meet Chloe in a public place so he could put a definite end to her obsession. Their meeting place was a restaurant of Chloe's choice. She instructed the chef, who was a close friend of hers, to make a special appetizer which was loaded with aphrodisiacs. Still, Brian was not attracted to Chloe. Instead, he was abrupt, stern, and to the point. He made it clear that he wanted nothing to do with her. After their meeting, he changed all his phone lines to unlisted numbers, canceled his e-mail account, and moved to a building with a better security system.

In spite of all this, Chloe was even more encouraged, simply because Brian had actually agreed to meet her. She saw it as their first date. In her excitement, she decided to prepare meals for Brian and have them delivered to his office. She spiked the offerings with aphrodisiac ingredients and performed a ritual over them to enchant him. She believed she had the power to put a spell on him, but Brian always sent the meals back untouched.

Chloe invited friends over to increase the power of her *Brian Rituals*. After her ceremony, she would go around in a circle with a crystal wand, point at each person, and ask them for their prediction of a wedding date.

Her friends thought of Chloe as somewhat of a celebrity, but they soon began to lose respect for her once they noticed her obsessive compulsive behavior. Every time a friend pointed out that Chloe might be stalking Brian or that Brian did not seem at all interested in her, she would disconnect from them in a harsh manner.

Over the years Chloe continued to find new ways to encroach on Brian's life. During this time, he dated many other women. He was very honest with her whenever she would send a message through a courier or follow him after he left his office, but she remained certain they would eventually be together. Twenty-one years passed, and Chloe did not veer once, and neither did Brian.

As Chloe's last attempt to elicit Brian's love, she called his office and left a long weepy message on the business machine, informing him that she would be in surgery on a certain day and that she did not think she could pull through unless Brian stood by her side. Brian never showed up. At the time, he was engaged to another woman, and he wanted help disconnecting from Chloe once and for all. He feared that he had somehow contributed to her lingering obsession because of his lack of firmness. His fiancé had been working with The Witnessing Technique, so she brought him in for a session.

When Brian showed up for his appointment, he was very open and willing to look into his programming. He quickly discovered a timid character in his mind which forced him to have limited boundaries with aggressive people. As the *witness*, Brian was able to construct firm and healthy boundaries without feeling guilty or frightened when confronted by dominating behavior.

After his fifth session, Brian wrote Chloe a very stern and to the point document, informing her that he was seeking a restraining order against her and that if she came within five hundred yards of his presence, he would press charges. She was also legally banned from calling his office. Brian left Chloe's life forever and set her free.

Chloe received the letter and was still upbeat. She was certain that Brian would see the light someday. A friend mentioned to Chloe that Brian had been practicing The Witnessing Technique, and she felt that her attendance might bring them closer together. She scheduled a session immediately.

When Chloe arrived for her appointment, she wanted to know if Brian had called asking if she had started therapy and what he had said. When she was informed that he had not called, her whole mood dropped into an angry, childlike brooding. Her tumultuous emotions created a powerful opportunity to begin the technique. Chloe was guided to allow her anger to form into an image, and the vision of an ugly, wicked witch with a big black wart on her nose and a big black crooked hat appeared in her mind. The witch was casting spells and boiling gooey green liquid in a steaming cauldron.

Chloe was certain that the witch was a vision of the girl Brian was about to marry. She thought she was having a psychic breakthrough, because Brian needed her to save him. Chloe was guided to watch the image until she felt neutral about it. When she closed her eyes again, however, the image pointed its crooked finger at her. *This is unusual, but often the character will acknowledge the observer, as the image itself is communication from the sub-conscious mind.* With this gesture, Chloe's anger ignited with a vengeance. She stood up and began tossing pillows about the room. Once she had settled down, she was guided to continue watching the image as though it were a movie. She sat down, closed her eyes, and eventually shared that the image was continuing to add ingredients to her cauldron. She stirred her potions, paced the dark steamy room, and wrung her wretched shriveled hands, all the while staring back at Chloe in her mind. Then she picked up a wand and began blasting everything in sight.

In horror, Chloe described how bad the witch appeared. Then she admitted that she had always feared that she might be a bad person. After fifteen minutes of observing the image, Chloe was able to see clearly that Brian's fiancée was not the witch. *Her vision was a representation of the programming which made Chloe believe that she was bad.* Chloe finally understood why she had such a strong need to prove that she was good and lovable. She left her appointment feeling dumfounded, but less clouded by her old mental programming.

When she returned for her next session, she shared that she had been having a recurring nightmare that her parents were condemning her. She had always wanted to prove to her parents that she was good and lovable, but they had disconnected from her when she refused to be a part of their fundamental church. Chloe also shared that she was still having difficulty identifying with her *Witnessing Self*, which is common when an obsessive mind tries to hold on to its goal.

Chloe was then asked how she felt about spending her life yearning for Brian without ever engaging in a relationship with him, and she immediately began to cry. Then she became angry and shouted that no one had any proof that Brian did not love her. Chloe was guided to allow her feelings to form into an image, and the vision of the witch appeared again. She was bubbling another brew, casting wicked spells, and looking around her den for ingredients to use in her potions. After watching this behavior for an extended period of time, Chloe finally felt neutral about the witch. Then she was guided to become aware of the aspect of her consciousness that was able to observe the image. Once Chloe had identified with her *Witnessing Self*, she let out a big sigh and expressed that she felt compassion for the character. She knew that the witch would be brewing potions for eternity, unaware of how powerless she was to make her spells come true.

As Chloe's *Witnessing Self* strengthened, the control her programming had over her began to diminish, and she was able to admit that she had never truly loved Brian. He represented a perfect combination of her distant mother and emotionless father. Her unhealed yearning to be acknowledged as good and lovable emerged simply because he symbolized her parents so intimately.

As Chloe identified more with her *Witnessing Self,* she developed a deep knowing that she was lovable and worthwhile. Although she dipped into her longing for Brian every few days at first, she finally realized that her obsession always caused her intense pain. As the *witness,* she felt free, powerful, and joyful. These feelings eventually became her healthy replacement for the intoxicating ones she longed to get from her obsessive thoughts. Once she made this conscious shift, she neither tried to contact Brian again, nor did she want to. She was finally free from her longing and pain.

Witnessing: A Path to Overcome
Service Obsession

Dom and Bertha worked together as nurses at a large hospital. They were in love and had been talking about marriage for three years. Dom was ready to plan the wedding and send out invitations, but Bertha had one main hurdle with Dom, which she was unable to overcome. When they were out on the road together, he would stop to help anyone who appeared to be in need of assistance. No matter what time of day or night it was, and no matter where they were headed, he would pull over. Often he would spend hours driving people to get gas, recharging batteries, or changing flat tires. He did all this without ever asking Bertha how she felt or what she wanted. His service to others also occurred while he was driving her to work, which caused her to arrive late on many occasions.

Most people suffering from Service Obsession will devote their lives to a partner or their children, consciously giving up their own happiness to make sure their loved ones have what they need. In Dom's case, however, he felt driven to devote himself to every victim in sight. To many people this may sound saint-like, but inevitably, the Service Obsessed builds resentment when great accolades of applause, recognition or retribution do not follow.

One night Bertha became sick after eating some bad food at a restaurant. Dom was quite concerned about Bertha as he was driving her to the hospital, but when he noticed a stranded motorist along the side of the road, he pulled over to help. Bertha stepped out of the car while she was having convulsions and fell into a ditch, but neither Dom nor the stranded motorist noticed. The motorist Dom rescued happened to be a healthy businessman, who had already called AAA auto emergency services to assist him. He told Dom he did not need his help, but Dom insisted on being his savior.

When Dom found Bertha she was unconscious in the ditch. He rushed her to the nearest hospital, and the doctors worked on her for quite a while, pumping her stomach while trying to counteract the effects of the reaction she had experienced. When Bertha became conscious two hours later, Dom was nowhere to be seen. At the time, he was in the parking lot reprimanding another visitor for leaving his dog in the car with only two windows rolled down. Dom felt he had to save the dog and punish the owner; even though the dog was in no danger, because it was a cool evening.

Bertha was furious with Dom for abandoning her, but in his mind, his heroic actions had saved yet another stranded motorist and a dog. Dom neither offered an apology, nor did he see any reason to do so. Bertha told him she never wanted to see him again unless he went through therapy to find out why he always had to rescue everyone in sight. Dom refused, stating that if anyone needed therapy it was Bertha, because she only cared about herself.

Dom walked out of Bertha's life that day. He began dating many of the other nurses at the hospital, but all the women he dated had the same problem with him. Dom still loved Bertha, so he agreed to come in for a Witnessing session. However, he made it clear to Bertha that he still did not believe he had a problem, and he was only doing it for her.

Dom found it difficult to find a time for an appointment, because his schedule was packed with volunteer work and fund raising for charities. He was adamant about getting in to please Bertha, so a special arrangement was made for a lunch hour session. Dom was informed that if he needed to change or cancel his appointment, twenty-four-hour notice would be required. He agreed to all the conditions and took down the address.

When the day for Dom's appointment arrived, he showed up for his one hour session forty-five minutes late, explaining that he had seen a homeless person on the side of the road and decided to take him out for lunch. Dom looked very proud of himself and waited for a pat on the back for being such a good citizen. No response was given in order to allow his programming to surface. When applause did not materialize, he appeared offended and angry. He shut down, crossed his arms, and stared indignantly out of the window. Dom was asked to express his feelings, but instead he spent the rest of the session defending his sacrosanct self-image, determined to prove his righteousness.

When Dom arrived for his second scheduled appointment he was punctual, but he refused to begin the session until he had recounted all the good deeds he had done for everyone he had come across throughout the day. After his fifteen minute narrative, he had a huge smile on his face, expecting some form of standing ovation. No response was given in order to allow his programming to be felt. When comments of appreciation did not follow, Dom once again became angry and acted as if he had been deeply offended. He shut down, crossed his arms, and thrust his lower lip out in a childish pout.

Dom was then asked what sort of a response he was hoping to elicit with his detailed description of all his helpful deeds, and he shared that he deserved a medal for being such a good person. In fact, he felt that he was the only good person with feelings and compassion left on the planet. When asked how this made him feel, he blurted out that it made him feel alone.

He was guided to allow his feelings to take the form of an image, and the vision of an old refugee woman with torn and tattered clothing appeared in his mind. He went on to describe her as worthless and unlovable, because she was a bad person, who had never really loved anyone in her life.

As he continued to watch the character, he noticed that she was searching for some way to redeem herself. She had big bulging eyes, and she was seeking someone who would look at her and give her another chance. No one would come near her, so she forced herself on others by tearing off pieces of her clothing and handing them out to whoever passed by, hoping they would see that she was trying. When no one was around to accept her rags, she became frantic and searched for additional ways to prove that she was good and lovable.

Dom was guided to connect with the aspect of his consciousness that was able to observe the image, and he immediately recognized the programming as a need to make up for some perceived fault within his own being. He reached out to people for affirmation of who he was, relying on others and the good deeds he could perform, as a way to prove to himself that he was a good person.

As he continued to practice The Witnessing Technique, he uncovered many more images within his psyche which caused him to believe he was unworthy and bad, unless he saved, healed, and reformed the planet. Once he had more practice identifying with Pure Consciousness, he realized that his *Witnessing Self* was his authentic self, and that he was innately good, even if he never rescued another person.

Dom also recognized how innocent Bertha was and how unloving his actions had been toward her. In his quest to serve others, he had not been honoring Bertha or many of his other commitments. Bertha and Dom both practice The Witnessing Technique, and they are seeing more eye to eye about what is appropriate and what is not when it comes to helping others. Their relationship no longer suffers from their old dispute, and the plans for their wedding are back on.

Witnessing: A Path to Overcome
Social Climber Obsession

Amos was an insecure middle-aged man who flaunted false wealth and only dated remarkably gorgeous women as a means to boost his social status. He was obsessed not with the women themselves, but with their beauty and what they could do for his reputation. In his mind, a woman's only purpose was to make him feel important, and he was indignant when they were not willing to appease his self-absorbed desires. He also expected complete devotion from his conquests, but he was far from monogamous himself. He searched every party for a more beautiful woman to top the one with whom he had arrived, and made a point of leaving with her instead.

When Amos met Ginger he was more obsessed than ever to mold her into his dream girl. Instead, Ginger recognized his motivation and suggested that he make an appointment to practice The Witnessing Technique. He agreed, hoping that would convince her to accept a date with him.

When Amos called for his session, he shared that the most painful emotion he experienced with his beautiful girls was the feeling of not being important enough for them to want to change for him. When Amos was guided to close his eyes and allow his feelings to form into an image, the vision of a meek, pimply-faced teenager with a mallet in his hand appeared. The teenager was walking around clubbing anyone who would not support his emotional needs.

Amos named the teenager Boyd and described him as unattractive, angry, and insecure. Boyd had to prove to everyone that he was important and worthy of attention, so he waved his mallet around and tried to control people with fear. After he had finished beating people, he appeared shorter, less significant, uglier, and more ridiculous.

Amos admitted that Boyd reminded him a bit of himself as a teenager. He had been a very unpopular and unattractive youth, and girls never paid attention to him. He wanted to punish beautiful girls, because he perceived them as shallow and assumed they chose their boyfriends based on good looks and social status. Whenever Amos treated a beautiful woman as a discardable object, he could feel the angry teenager inside of himself taking his revenge.

Amos was guided to connect with the aspect of his consciousness that was able to observe the image, but he had a lot of resistance. He ended the session abruptly, declaring that he would prove that all women were interested in were good-looking men with social status.

After three months of physical transformation, Amos felt quite proud of his new appearance, so he called Ginger and invited himself over to see her. When he arrived at her house, however, all his insignificant programming came rushing back. He realized that his insecurities were buried much deeper than he thought. Not knowing what else to do, he came in for another appointment.

Amos spent the first fifteen minutes expressing his anger toward Ginger for making him feel insignificant. Then he was guided to close his eyes and allow his anger to form into an image. To his surprise, the same image of Boyd with his mallet appeared. This time, however, Amos allowed himself to identify with the aspect of his consciousness that was able to observe the insignificant character, and he instantly experienced a profound sense of inner confidence. As the *witness*, he felt at peace in a way he had never imagined possible, and he finally understood that he had to feel good about himself from the inside, no matter what others thought about him on the outside.

From that point forward, whenever Amos felt the urge to possess or manipulate a beautiful woman, he remembered the image of Boyd and quickly identified with his *Witnessing Self* instead. Once he felt empowered and whole from within, his relationships became much more fulfilling, and he no longer felt the need to use a beautiful woman to boost his ego or social image.

Witnessing: A Path to Overcome
Unrequited Obsession

Tanya grew up in a grand Hollywood home. Her parents were in the industry, and they expected great things from her. In her mind, she had chosen the movie star she would marry so that she could carry on with her Hollywood status. She had also picked out her wedding dress, her wedding ring, and the house she wanted her future movie star husband to buy for her. Tanya went through the motions of dating many boys, but she never allowed herself to take much interest in them. She dreamt of the day when all her ex-boyfriends would see her in magazines holding hands with her movie star husband.

On Tanya's twenty-second birthday, her mother threw a big party for her at their Hollywood home and invited many celebrities; including the movie star with whom she had been obsessed since she was a teen. When the party began, and the star appeared, she ran to her room in tears. Her mother came in to speak with her, but she refused to return to the party.

The next day Tanya's mother suggested she begin therapy to see what was holding her back from her ultimate success, so Tanya decided to come in for a Witnessing session. When she arrived she was vivacious, upbeat, and very open about her history with men. Eventually she was asked to share what emotion had been evoked when her "Celebrity Love" entered her birthday party. She admitted that she felt terrified he would reject her.

Tanya was guided to allow the feeling of being rejected to form into an image, and the vision of a monster creature appeared in her mind. The monster was slimy and fish-like, and it reminded her of the character *Gollum* from Lord of the Rings, so she named the character "Miss Gollum." Miss Gollum did not believe she would ever be wanted by anyone. She instead chose power over people without their knowledge. While hidden in her cave, she would watch others and visualize various ways of manipulating them.

Tanya wanted to choreograph Miss Gollum and redeem her from her sins by transforming the ugly image into something more pleasant, so she was reminded that the image was just a program in her mind. The more she wanted to change the image to her liking, the more identified she would become with it. Tanya understood and went home intent on observing the character without trying to improve her.

When Tanya arrived for her next session, she was detached enough from the image to recognize that it was a program in her mind. It represented her core fears of being unwanted and unworthy of love. She feared that anyone who had expectations of her disguised self would be disappointed by her undisguised self.

As Tanya continued practicing The Witnessing Technique, her "movie star" obsession faded. It had all been a fantasy in her mind to hide her fear of being unwanted. Her obsession had also kept her from diving into real love with men she dated. Once she rose above her programming, she no longer needed to live in the safety zone of Unrequited Obsession. She finally felt ready to experience true intimacy.

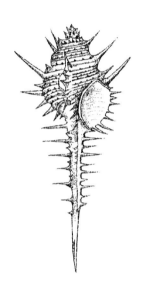

CHAPTER 11

Panic Attacks

Introduction

Sudden overwhelming terror that overpowers thoughts, emotions, and physical responses in an aggressive way.

FOR MOST PEOPLE, SAFETY AND STABILITY are arrived at solely through material structures, such as the comfort received through a family unit or support group, a parental figure or mentor, a bank account, loyal friends, a committed partner, a successful career, time, attention, health, youth, physical attractiveness, outer peace, consistency, and familiarity. When these outside structures and securities fall away or become untrustworthy, anxiety leading into panic is often the result.

Many people depend on a belief system, religious devotion, or political conviction for their safety structure. If any flaw appears in their system, or if it is challenged by a powerful force, a deep feeling of insecurity will arise as well.

Stress

Stress is a leading factor in elevated levels of anxiety, which can culminate in panic. A move to another country, financial loss, career uncertainty, a break-up, health issues, extreme exhaustion, deadlines, excessive travel, odd hours, abrupt change, too much diversity, shock, unexpected loss, or the death of someone who represented strength, security, or structure, can trigger core fears and cause a panic attack.

All anxieties arise due to a lack of connection to an inner source of strength and stability one can lean on when all outside sources fail. Once an individual learns to depend on their *Witnessing Self*, they will no longer experience panic attacks, anxiety, or compulsive fear. Solid, everlasting stability and strength will only arise through a deep connection with Pure Consciousness.

Witnessing: A Path to Overcome

Panic Due to Loss

Originally from England, Liam followed his brother to America to help him build a children's clothing empire. After five years in their new location, Liam's brother; who had been a father figure to him since the age of six, died and left him to run the company alone. His pillar of strength and security no longer existed.

Soon after the death of his brother, Liam discovered that one of his employees had embezzled over two hundred thousand dollars worth of merchandise. In order to make up this loss, Liam doubled his work efforts by taking on his brother's prior business obligations, and began traveling to shows and markets throughout Europe. One night in Turkey, Liam happened to step into a store run by brothers, and suddenly his heart seized up.

At first he thought he was having a heart attack, because he was unable to breathe, and he had shooting pain in his chest. He also felt faint and overwhelmed, as if he might pass out or be sick to his stomach. The merchants in the store came to his assistance, and within thirty minutes Liam was breathing almost normally, and his physical distress had subsided. He was shaken up and worried about what had happened, but he had no further episodes while he was in Turkey.

After a brief rest, Liam embarked upon an even more rigorous plan of travel for his company. Spending only one night in each town, he made his way through Italy, Greece, and France. After two weeks of traveling, he walked into a small shop in Paris and suddenly his panic re-emerged. He broke into a sweat, turned ghost white, and grabbed his chest—although his pain seemed to be coming from somewhere intangible. Liam went to see a doctor who suggested that he may have experienced a panic attack. He put him on anti-anxiety pills and told him to stay away from caffeine.

While back in the States, Liam had no further attacks, but on his third trip that year, he once again found himself collapsing in horror as panic enveloped his body and mind, and he thought he was dying. When he returned home, he changed doctors three times and started therapy to help with his emotions, but the panic felt even closer to the surface as his fear of having another attack grew.

Months went by just waiting for the next attack, when finally it happened on a plane to London. Liam was booked in business class, but he arrived late and was given a coach seat in the back of the plane. The air was poor, the ride was bumpy, and he was wedged in the middle seat between two rather heavy passengers. When the dinner cart passed by and blocked the aisle way, Liam's heart jumped into his throat. He felt suspended, hovering in the midst of a nightmare while his energy was being sucked out in the most painful and horrifying manner. He shot out of his seat clutching his chest and escaped into the bathroom, where he spent the remainder of the flight.

Desperate to find a cure, Liam took time off to research panic attacks himself, hoping to gain control over his situation. He received acupuncture, massage, and reflexology, and he started taking calming herbs. Nonetheless, his terror over having another panic attack continued. His acupuncturist recommended The Witnessing Technique, and he agreed to come in for a session.

When Liam arrived, he shared that his most intense emotion was terror, so he was guided to allow his terror to form into an image. The vision of a man standing on the edge of a crumbling jetty appeared. It seemed that at any moment he would lose his bearings and plummet into the abyss. As long as Liam watched the teetering man, however, he never actually fell. Instead, he simply stood in his precarious position hovering on the verge of faltering. The uncertainty felt unbearable. *Liam's programming caused him to feel there was no move he could make that would be safe. He was always on the verge of tumbling into an abyss. There seemed to be no safety, stability, or structure anywhere in his life.*

As soon as Liam felt neutral about the teetering image, he was guided to identify with the aspect of his consciousness that was able to observe the man on the cliff. Once he had identified with his *Witnessing Self,* he shared that he felt stable, secure, and peaceful as the *witness.* Even while he watched the precarious image on the cliff, his *Witnessing Self* remained strong, confident, and unaffected. When Liam slipped back into identifying with the teetering image, he felt a frightening sense of helplessness that he knew could lead to panic. Once he realized that he could choose to identify with either perspective, a deep calm settled within. He had options, and he only had to remain aware.

Liam was persistent and consistent with his Witnessing practice. Soon he found it easy to remain identified with the strong, safe, peaceful aspect of his consciousness that remained invincible and calm under all circumstances. Through all his diligence, Liam was able to rise above many of his old programmed fears within a few weeks of practicing the technique. For the first time since his brother had died, he felt a powerful sense of stability. This time, however, it was based on his inner strength, verses an outer support system. Once his fear of loss had evaporated, his panic never returned.

Witnessing: A Path to Overcome

Panic Due to Overwhelming Circumstances

Maria was a secretary at a busy firm. Her husband had been unemployed for two years, so she worked overtime as much as possible to make ends meet. On the weekends, she would complain about her minor aches and pains, and her husband would drink beer and listen until he fell asleep. This was the only bonding time they shared in their marriage.

One day Maria came home to find her husband in bed with another woman. She grabbed some personal belongings and went to a hotel. The next day she called in sick to work and went looking for an apartment. Maria searched for two weeks until she found a new home. Her boss was less than compassionate about all the time she had missed, but Maria was beyond caring about her job. She was only trying to make it through each day.

When Maria went back to work miserable and moody, she discovered that her archenemy had been put in charge of her division while she was gone. Her replacement had also been doing a better job than Maria had, according to her boss, so Maria was laid off two weeks later.

On her way home from her last day of work, Maria's heart jumped into her throat, and her stomach seized up. She was suddenly dizzy and perspiring profusely, and she felt herself losing control of her bodily functions. She rushed to her new apartment building, but she was unable to make it all the way to her door in time. Her clothes were ruined, and she felt humiliated in the hallway in front of her new neighbors.

Maria sat in the bathroom all night with a nervous stomach. She had diarrhea and a headache, as well as a racing petrified feeling in her heart. The next day she felt physically better, so she decided to keep an interview she had set up for a new job. When she entered the large office building, the same unnerving anxiousness arose. She raced around searching for a bathroom, but was unable to find one. She collapsed in pain and shame in the middle of the office building, clasping at her heart and stomach. The paramedics were called, but all the tests performed at the hospital determined that she was in perfect health.

Maria went home and cried herself to sleep. She waited a week before she convinced herself she felt ready to venture out again, but when her next interview date arrived, her chest suddenly seized up as she stepped outside of her apartment door. She fell to the ground and crawled back inside to the bathroom, quivering with terror.

Maria stopped scheduling job interviews and instead began interviewing doctors to find out what could be causing her trouble. She was certain that her loss of control had to be biological, because she had such severe physical symptoms. Each doctor she visited, however, found nothing wrong with her body. After giving up on doctors, Maria discovered ways to live within the confines of her safe apartment by doing her banking over the internet and having her groceries delivered. As time progressed, however, her physical symptoms multiplied. She began to swell, her feet hurt, and she could not sit for more than ten minutes without her back seizing up in pain. Her glands were sore, her joints were aching, and her vision was blurry. The list continued to grow as she needed more reasons to validate her desire to stay home.

One day Maria woke up with a severe tooth ache. She was unable to find a dentist that would come to her, so she was forced to leave her apartment. She had three mini panic attacks on the way to the dentist's office, but she was able to calm herself down enough to arrive safely. After the dentist did what he could with her tooth, she discovered that she would have to come back at least two more times to have the work completed properly.

Maria was devastated. Reality was hitting her hard. She was out of money, her body was falling apart quickly, and she realized she could not maintain her reclusive lifestyle much longer. In desperation, she called an old friend hoping that she could borrow money from him. Instead of agreeing to a loan, her friend mentioned The Witnessing Technique and offered to pay for her first five sessions. Maria respected him and felt willing to try. She made an appointment that day.

When Maria called for her session, she shared that she was sweating from head to toe, her chest was tight, and her stomach felt acidy. She seemed very attached to her physical maladies as she described them enthusiastically. Maria eventually shared that dread was the most intense feeling that arose for her right before her panic attacks. She was guided to allow this emotion to form into an image, and the vision of a very tense, bitter old woman with wrinkled skin and cigarette smoke smoldering all around her appeared. The woman looked haggard, so Maria named the image, "Haggard." Her emotions were being held inside her body, because she was too proud to allow others the satisfaction of seeing the emotional pain they had caused.

When Maria understood that the haggard character represented programming in her psyche, she was confused, because she had always been the strong one who had taken care of others. When all of her safety systems had fallen apart, however, she reverted into a quivering mass of fear. Life had brought her into an experience of pain far beyond her coping capabilities. She was overwhelmed and overloaded with stress.

Maria watched the image until she felt neutral. Then she was guided to connect with the aspect of her consciousness that was able to observe the character. Once she had identified with her *Witnessing Self,* she experienced a distinct shift in perspective. For the first time in years, she felt strong, confident, and healthy.

Maria practiced The Witnessing Technique each day until the Haggard character became easy to recognize within her. She gained total control over her bodily functions within the first month of practicing the technique, and recaptured her powerful vitality soon after. It took Maria almost three months to get back into a thriving routine of socializing, working, and feeling confident in public again, but she re-emerged with greater strength and happiness than she had ever known. In fact, Maria felt so good about herself and so positive about life that she was able to attract a very loving man, who happened to be extraordinarily wealthy. Once they married, Maria lived a life of creativity and luxurious travel with the man of her dreams.

CHAPTER 12

Phobias

Introduction

An irrational fear, hatred, or aversion to a specific object, stimulus, activity, person, or situation.

A PHOBIA CAN MANIFEST IN A NUMBER OF WAYS. The more complicated phobic mind will attempt to protect the self from a real fear, by superimposing an irrational fear of something which represents the true fear in its place. A small child who is traumatized by an event may tune out the pain in her body and soul and tune into the sound of music playing nearby. Once the trauma is superimposed onto the melody, the child can continue to feel relatively untouched by the event. In her mind, the event did not occur, the music did. The child has no way of knowing this consciously, because it has all been safely locked away deep within her subconscious. However, if this same melody is heard, even if it is fifty years later, she will experience unsettling feelings all over again, without any understanding of the root cause.

The trauma of an event can be projected onto anything: a scent, a sound, a vision, a touch, a person, a picture, a color, a culture, a gender, a simultaneous event, a season, a date, or a headache they had at the time. A painful experience does not necessarily have to be projected onto something which was present while the distress occurred. Often a traumatic event becomes symbolized by something which reminds the individual of his or her terror, such as an animal, character, or weather condition.

When a phobia is triggered, it will activate a highly accentuated level of panic or hatred in relation to the actual threat or danger present. Those most susceptible to phobias are generally extremely sensitive or mentally dependent individuals, who are more vulnerable and tuned into the mind's working mechanism and response signals. Therefore, they are more likely to identify with the mind and give it total control over their reactions to life.

Less problematic phobias, such as stepping over cracks in the sidewalk or the need for extreme cleanliness are common. The ego has simply found a ritual to apply in order to feel protected from the real fear that the mind has suppressed. If these rituals are not completed, an intense dread that something unbearable, overpowering, or uncomfortable, will subsequently occur. A strong connection to the *Witnessing Self* is all that is needed to overcome phobias. Once identification with Pure Consciousness has been established, one can easily rise above the mind where all displacement and phobic fear reside.

Witnessing: A Path to Overcome
The Phobic Mind

Audrey had a phobic fear of sharks. Her fear began at the age of three and increased in its intensity as she grew. Not only was she petrified of the ocean, but she also refused to swim in pools and lakes. When she turned nine, she became too frightened to step into bath water, fearing that a shark would somehow enter the bathtub and attack her. Even though Audrey had never watched any shark movies, and she had never seen any pictures of shark attacks, she was terrified of them nonetheless.

Because of her fear, Audrey refused to fly over any body of water—a situation that became a very big challenge for her when she turned twenty-five and fell in love. Her boyfriend was an avid traveler and wanted to take her all over the world. Audrey thought that perhaps her love for Luke would help her overcome her phobia of sharks, but whenever he spoke of travel plans, she would shut down or change the subject.

One weekend Luke arranged a romantic get-away to Lake Tahoe. He agreed to drive just so that Audrey would not have to fly over any water. They enjoyed a candlelight dinner their first evening, and then Luke turned on the hot tub and jumped in. He had no idea that Audrey would be afraid of sharks in the jacuzzi, so when she refused to come in, he picked her up and threw her in as a joke. Audrey went into a panic and began to scream, so Luke pulled her out and put her to bed. That was the end of their romantic weekend. Luke drove Audrey home the next day and told her that she needed to see a psychiatrist.

Audrey knew her fear of finding a shark in a jacuzzi was irrational, but she was unable to contain her terror. She was concerned that a psychiatrist may indeed find that she was crazy, so when a friend suggested The Witnessing Technique as an alternative, she made an appointment.

The thought of a shark inspired unprecedented terror for Audrey. She was guided to allow her emotion to form into an image, and the vision of a child in a dark room appeared in her mind. The child lay very still and silent because she was frightened of what might happen if anyone knew she was there. Something was lurking in the dark, but she did not know what it was. Audrey agreed to observe the image during the week and pay attention to anything unusual that appeared in her thoughts and emotions.

When Audrey arrived for her next session, she was eager to talk about a recurring nightmare that she had been having since her first session. In the dream she was swimming in the ocean with her brother. Within moments a shark would appear and swim right over to Audrey and rip her apart. The shark never touched her brother. He always swam safely back to shore, leaving Audrey with the shark.

Audrey was asked if this reminded her of anything. She thought for a moment, and then answered that her grandfather had beaten her quite badly all the way up until she was thirteen, but that he had never touched her brother. Her brother was the grandfather's favorite child, and he was praised for everything he did. Audrey on the other hand, was always hiding behind corners afraid that her grandfather would attack her for no reason at all.

After Audrey expressed this, she inhaled sharply and realized what she had uncovered. The shark was her grandfather. He was unpredictable and vicious. He would rip her apart verbally and attack her physically, leaving her immobile and injured afterwards. Her grandfather did not seem to need a reason to attack her, and sometimes he would hide in rooms and jump on her when she least expected it. When Audrey told her parents about this they accused her of lying. In fact, when she told her father, he slapped her across the face with such fury, that he gave her a black eye. Audrey was so traumatized by these events that she began to believe there was no safe place on earth for her. Even her brother attacked her once he discovered that her accusations were not taken seriously.

Audrey was shocked to realize that she had carried the memory of the abuse around with her as a phobia, without putting the pieces together. Her mind had tricked her so well that she believed she was more afraid of sharks than she was of her grandfather. A shark was the most unpredictable, lurking-in-the-dark symbol that her mind could have chosen.

Audrey spent many of her sessions becoming aware of numerous images all formed due to her core fear of being unsafe. She observed all of the images until she felt a neutral sensation about them and her fear, rage, and pain quickly transformed into relief, freedom, and compassion. As the *witness*, she reconnected with her personal power, which brought her a sense of safety under all conditions. Audrey is now free to enjoy the great adventures of the ocean and taking a bath has become one of her favorite forms of relaxation.

Witnessing: A Path to Overcome
Multiple Phobias

Although Joey and Billy were twins, they were not at all alike. Joey was quiet, introverted, and creative. Billy was boisterous, extroverted, and destructive. Billy thrived on getting attention, and Joey preferred to be alone and go unnoticed.

Whenever Joey became the center of positive attention, Billy would find ways to sabotage his brother in order to make him appear bad. A common tactic he employed was breaking something of importance and blaming it on Joey, who would be caught off-guard and only later discover why he had been punished. Joey neither argued nor stood up for himself, because he feared Billy's vengeance.

When the twins entered school, Billy made it his mission to cause disharmony between Joey and his friends, so that Joey would not appear more popular. After one very humiliating situation Billy had orchestrated, Joey began waking up screaming in the middle of the night. He was unable to keep food down and he started losing his hair. He was experiencing extremely high levels of emotional, mental, and physical stress. As his fear of Billy increased, he started obsessing over the worst case scenarios his brother could create for him, and his mind began to race ahead frantically searching for a way to protect himself.

Suddenly Joey became afraid of wearing yellow or brown clothing. His fear intensified to such an extreme, that when his mother purchased yellow or brown outfits for him, he would throw himself on the bed crying. Joey's lack of gratitude for the clothing made him appear selfish and spoiled, and he was punished for his behavior. Meanwhile, Billy was enjoying the whole situation, because he was appearing more and more as the good twin.

One day Joey was running away from Billy in an abandoned logging facility, when he stepped on a nail which went right through his shoe into his foot. The trauma of the injury set off an array of new phobias, all of which revolved around the fear of being invaded. Suddenly, he was unable to watch television without having a phobic response. If there was an unappealing character on the television screen and someone called Joey's name, he thought he would turn into the unappealing image. The thought petrified Joey. He did not know how it started or how to stop it and he couldn't explain why he went into a fit when the television was turned on.

Soon Joey became afraid of stepping on the cracks in the sidewalk. In his mind, any negative thought would immediately manifest itself if he stepped on a crack at the same time that he was thinking a negative thought. He did not trust that he could project a positive thought simultaneously with his foot placement, because his mind had complete control over him.

Joey also had difficulty writing his name on his assignments at school. If he was writing his name and someone said something negative, he was frightened that he would take on the negativity. His teacher perceived Joey's behavior as defiant and sent him to the principal's office regularly, where he would receive a detention.

Each year an additional set of phobias would enter his psyche. When he turned twelve, Joey became afraid that if he rode his bicycle around the block clockwise, he would have to ride his bike around the block counter-clockwise, or he would end up in a different world or a different reality like the Twilight Zone. Terrified, he would retrace his tracks exactly, in an attempt to counteract his phobic anxiety and keep his mind from going into a panic.

When Joey graduated from high school, he left home immediately and moved to another city five thousand miles away. He changed his name, put on fifteen needed pounds, and took a job as a produce manager at a local market. The move was very good for him, and he was surprised to discover that many of his phobias disappeared almost immediately. He made new friends and even found a wonderful girl he enjoyed dating.

Everyone liked Joey in his new town, and he became quite popular. For the first time in his life he was not withdrawn or reclusive. He was involved with sports and social events, and he went out on weekends with his friends. He was a completely different person. After nine months of blissful existence in his new town, Joey's grandmother passed away. He went back to stay with his family for one week, and all of his phobias came rushing back with even greater force.

When Joey returned to his own house he was withdrawn and elusive. His girlfriend noticed the change in him and felt that it had something to do with his family visit. Joey was not ready to tell his girlfriend about his phobias, but he did feel safe with her. When she suggested The Witnessing Technique, he agreed to come in for a session.

When Joey arrived he was very pleasant, thoughtful, receptive, and eager to apply everything that was offered. When it came time to express, however, he clammed up and appeared petrified. He fidgeted, and blushed the shade of crimson. Following an uncomfortable pause, he made an excuse that he had to leave immediately and bolted out of the office.

Surprisingly, Joey showed up for his next session. He apologized for leaving so abruptly the time before, then shared that he was ready to tell someone the truth about what was happening in his mind. He confided the long list of phobias with which he had struggled. Then he shared that his current trauma had to do with wearing yellow or brown clothing, which happened to be the color of his mandatory coveralls at work. He feared that if he wore yellow or brown, Billy would have the power to make something terrible happen, like a witch doctor with a voodoo doll. He was still petrified of Billy five thousand miles away.

Joey was guided to close his eyes. He allowed his fear to form into an image, and the vision of a small ball of clay appeared. The clay had been manipulated and formed into many different objects and lay scrunched up and vulnerable on a table. He was afraid someone very bad would pick it up and turn it into something that the clay did not want to be, because it had no way to protect itself and no way of knowing what was going to happen to it next.

Joey was guided to identify with his *Witnessing Self* and describe his experience from that perspective. He was quiet for a long while, as a beautiful expression formed slowly on his face. He said that he felt powerful, safe, and in control of his life for the first time. He could see clearly from the *witnessing* position that he was not the clay. He was the powerful observer of the programming, and he *did* have the strength to protect himself. The clay only represented a belief in his mind that he was vulnerable and easily molded into anything Billy wanted him to be. As the *witness*, he saw no reason to fear Billy. Joey had tears of joy in his eyes when he left that day. He was discovering his true power, and that felt good.

When Joey arrived for his next session, he was like a young boy; playful, talkative, and exuberant. He shared the insights he had been having and said he was beginning to feel as though he had authority over his mind. However, Joey wanted to work on one phobia in particular that seemed to resist his *Witnessing* attempts. The phobia with which Joey was having difficulty came up whenever he would see an unpleasant or disturbing sight, such as an ambulance rushing to a scene, animal excrement on the ground, a homeless person passed out under a bench, or someone's angry face. If he saw one of these scenes as someone called out his name, he believed that he would take on the energy of the scene or fall into danger. The emotion this brought up for him was petrified fear.

Joey closed his eyes and allowed his feelings to form into an image, and the vision of a small boy without any center appeared. The boy was empty inside. He had no guts. Because he was empty, anything could enter him. All he had to do was think of something or see something, and he would become contaminated. He kept running away, hoping to escape anything that could possess him or take him over energetically. Joey worked himself into a frenzy as he described the image. He was frightened that what he said was true, and that he was vulnerable to anything and everything just by looking at it or thinking about it. *He understood the power of his thoughts, but he did not know how to wield them.*

When Joey was guided to become aware of the aspect of his consciousness that was able to observe the image, he visibly relaxed and took a deep breath. He shared that the boy in his image was empty, because he did not know himself. Distinguishing himself as the *witness*, would not only give him a powerful identity, it would help him remain in his own center.

Eventually, Joey recognized that his programming seemed to be covering up his *core fear* of being *powerless*; the basis of all his phobias. Joey could ride his bicycle counter-clockwise around the block or isolate himself from others, but he had no tools to deal with the helplessness he experienced around his brother. Therefore, his mind intervened, offering him symbolic fears of which he *did* feel in control.

As Joey continued to practice the Technique, miraculous things began to happen for him. He grew two inches at the age of twenty-one, his eye sight improved so much that he no longer had the need for glasses, and all of his allergies disappeared. He went back to school to become a research scientist. He graduated with honors, and he ran a marathon, finishing in the top twenty.

Once Joey felt safe applying his power, he was able to reach his true potential. He married his long-time girlfriend, and they both practice The Witnessing Technique to work through any challenges that come up in their relationship. Joey also finds time to visit with his family, since they can no longer affect him negatively. He understands how to remain strong and confident as the *witness*.

CHAPTER 13

Relationships

Love

A Flowering of Pure Consciousness

WE RECEIVE A GLIMPSE OF PURE CONSCIOUSNESS during the initial phase of falling in love. Our energy literally falls from the mind into the heart. For this brief period the mind is bypassed, and the opportunity for a pure experience of life without the ego's influence is created. In essence, love offers an opening for us to know the bliss of our being.

During this euphoria, a beloved can do no wrong. Once the mind re-enters, however, by categorizing and fault finding, the habitual labeling of good-bad, right-wrong and true-false are re-established. These dichotomies create the love-hate of relationships.

The love we feel in a union reflects our true self
or Pure Consciousness. The pain we feel in a union
reflects our ego or programming.

To fulfill the longing for which we all yearn in love, we must move inward toward our source. The Witnessing Technique and The Love Meditation will make this simple as well as guide the way.

Witnessing: A Path to Overcome

Heartbreak

As long as we identify with the ego, the outer world holds the ability to control our thoughts, feelings, and reactions—allowing others to mold our identity. In relationships, we are more susceptible than ever to losing our center and falling prey to the agenda of those to whom we become attached, admire, or fear.

When Pearl met Suillus, she was at a high point in her life. She had just turned eighteen and signed with a big modeling agency in Chicago. Suillus was a Prince from another country doing business in Chicago for one year. He had an endearing presence, and Pearl thought she had found the man of her dreams. Three months into their relationship, Suillus proposed. Shortly after the wedding invitations had been sent out, however, Pearl discovered Suillus in bed with one of the other models from her agency. In his defense, Suillus listed all of Pearl's shortcomings, leaving her with a shattered self-image and a broken heart.

In the depths of her sorrow, a photographer approached Pearl and shared the emotional recovery he had experienced with The Witnessing Technique after his divorce, and Pearl made an appointment right away. When she called for her session, she was very clear that the most intense emotion she felt was rage, so she was guided to allow her emotion to form into an image, and the vision of a woman appeared. She was standing rigid with her arms and legs forcefully pressed together, and her anger was so hot that she eventually burst into flames. Once Pearl had reached a neutral feeling about the image, she was guided to connect with the aspect of her consciousness that was able to observe the character. She identified with her *Witnessing Self* easily and immediately felt removed from her pain.

As the session continued, Pearl expressed interest in rising above her fear of being vulnerable. She was invited to allow her feelings to form into an image, and the vision of an angelic looking child appeared. Engulfed in a white glowing light, she stood naïvely, looking around in wonder, trusting everything, open to everyone, totally unaware that others would be less angelic than herself. There was a pause on the phone and then Pearl began to cry. She shared that she felt unsafe living in the world among so many unscrupulous people who had no heart. She wanted to protect the child and save her from harm's way. Instead, she was guided to detach and observe the image as a symbol which represented her programming. She was able to recognize that she was not the angelic child who needed to be protected and saved. She was the powerful *witness*. Her *Witnessing Self* was also angelic and loving, but at the same time it was strong and self-reliant. Pearl was beginning to understand the difference between her old programmed idea of romantic love and living with awareness.

Once Pearl's anger had transformed, she was guided to open her heart to the love she felt for her puppy. Overflowing with the euphoria love brings, she found the source of her rapture located within her own body. Pearl was guided to embrace this beautiful feeling, acknowledging that all the love she needed could be found deep within. She would never have to look outside of her "self" for love again. Pearl continued to practice The Witnessing Technique every time she felt her mind move into painful thoughts or feelings. She applied The Love Meditation, using her puppy for inspiration, every night before she went to sleep.

As her inner healing evolved, Pearl's hatred and rage toward Suillus transformed into compassion, and within a few months she met a man who treated her with the love and respect for which she had always yearned. They were married twelve months later, and they practice The Witnessing Technique together to work through any conflicts that arise within their relationship.

Once we establish a strong connection with Pure Consciousness, our aware-ness will heighten, and the ability to make wise choices based on who we are and what brings us joy, will strengthen. From this higher perspective, we naturally gravitate toward those people and circumstances that prove uplifting and add to our bliss.

Witnessing: A Path to Overcome Abuse

When Clair first began working with The Witnessing Technique, she was in the most destructive relationship of her life. Her boyfriend beat her and threatened to kill her at least twice a month. At one point Claire had become pregnant with her boyfriend's baby. When she told him, he brutally attacked her and kicked her repeatedly in the abdomen in an attempt to abort the child. The fetus was not harmed in the assault, but Clair was knocked unconscious and suffered internal bleeding. When she awoke in the hospital, her boyfriend leaned over and whispered in her ear that if she kept the baby, he would kill her. She had an abortion, but she continued to have unprotected sex with her lover.

Recognizing that Clair was in an abusive relationship, a good friend suggested that she begin working with The Witnessing Technique. When she arrived, she shared that she felt helpless and incapable of leaving her abusive situation, but she feared she would certainly die if she remained. She was guided to close her eyes and allow her fear to form into an image. The vision of a tiny *baby Clair* appeared. The child was helpless, vulnerable, innocent, and powerless to protect herself in any way. All the needs of a child, such as love, tenderness, and attention, were not only absent, but also not expected. Clair had been programmed to live in instability, fear, and insecurity. Seeing this programming made her more aware of why she chose abusive relationships, and why she felt unable to leave them.

When she was invited to connect with the aspect of her consciousness that was able to observe the baby, she suddenly felt "capable" and in control of her life. Astonished by this sudden shift in perspective, she finished her session with a strong determination to remain connected to her *Witnessing Self* as much as possible during the week.

When Clair arrived for her next session she had a black eye. She had tried to cover it up with makeup and sunglasses, but openly admitted that she had been beaten by her boyfriend after taking a bold step forward to end her relationship with him. Her boyfriend went ballistic and threw her out of a window. For the first time, Clair filed a police report and attained a restraining order against him, which felt empowering for her.

The most painful emotion that had arisen for Clair during her ordeal, was the feeling of being discarded. She was guided to allow the intensity of her emotions to emerge as an image, and the vision of a five-year-old girl appeared. The girl was standing in a room with other people, but no one noticed her. She felt useless and without purpose, because she had nothing to offer. Clair suddenly gasped and shared that she had finally found a way to serve a purpose. She could be a punching bag or the *thing* upon which others used to vent their aggressions. That was the most she ever expected. To be loved would be too much to ask, because she believed she had no value.

Clair was guided to identify with the aspect of her consciousness that was able to observe the image. Once again she was shocked by her sudden shift in perspective. As the *witness*, she felt reverence for herself, and she finally realized that she was valid, even without serving some purpose for others. This drastic new perspective gave Clair great motivation and excitement to practice The Witnessing Technique daily in order to move beyond the horrific programming in her mind.

Clair spent two years getting to know herself from the *Witnessing* perspective, and when she began dating again, she was attracted to a completely different type of man. She felt exuberant to be treated with tenderness and respect. She is now guided from the higher awareness of her *Witnessing Self*, which honors and respects her at all times.

Witnessing: A Path to Overcome
Unhealthy Attraction

Bill and Claudia had been dating for six months. Claudia thought she loved Bill, but at the same time, she felt badly about herself whenever she was in his presence. Bill had a compulsive need for her attention, but he paid little or no attention to her.

Many times he would call her in a panic, pleading with her to come over right away. Claudia would rush over to his house, run up the steps, and ring the doorbell—only to be left waiting outside for up to ten minutes before he answered the door. After Bill finally opened the door, he would quickly disappear without any explanation and leave her standing in the entry way dumfounded. When he'd re-emerge ten to fifteen minutes later, he would pick up his cell phone and make two or three twenty-minute calls while she waited for him to finish. After his calls, he would log on the internet and check his e-mails while she sat patiently waiting. Bill never explained why he had called in a panic, desperate for her to be by his side. In fact, he always acted as though she had been uninvited. Claudia did not understand why, but she was intensely attracted to Bill and she continued to put up with his behavior.

After months of feeling unappreciated and unloved, Claudia decided she needed help disconnecting from her unhealthy attraction to Bill, and she scheduled a Witnessing session. The most painful emotion she felt at the time was the feeling of being ignored. She was guided to allow her feelings to form into an image, and the vision of a plastic-looking girl appeared. She neither looked real nor did she ever come into focus. *According to her programming, she did not really exist.*

Claudia was guided to identify with the aspect of her consciousness that was able to observe the image, and a powerful transformation occurred immediately. As the *witness*, she recognized that she had the right to have her own life, instead of living to boost other people's self-esteem. As a non-existent person, her dominant intent while interacting with others had always been to empower them, even if that meant diminishing herself.

As Claudia continued to practice The Witnessing Technique, she began to feel more legitimate as a person. The more valid she felt, the less interest she had in Bill. Within one week of identifying with her *Witnessing Self*, she was able to rise above her painful attraction to him once and for all.

When Claudia ended her relationship with Bill, he began calling her four or five times a day, showing up at her house unannounced, and sending flowers with love notes attached. Once she realized that he was not going to stop pursuing her, she gave him the contact number for The Witnessing Technique and told him that it might help. He made an appointment right away, assuming she would be encouraged to reconnect with him if he did so.

When Bill arrived, he shared that he felt abandoned and forgotten by Claudia, and that he did not think he could live without her. He was guided to close his eyes and allow his feelings to form into an image, and the vision of a nerdy kid with heavy black-rimmed glasses and a pimply face appeared. The kid was scrawny and insecure and he had a notebook in his hand, which he used to hide his face. Bill named the kid Jeffrey and went on to describe him as *a nobody*. He wanted to be *somebody*, but felt there was no way he could be. Consequently, he found girls who appeared to be *somebodies*, so he could demean them and in turn feel better about himself. Without Claudia in his life, he felt insignificant again, because he had no one to toy with or humiliate. He had no intention of treating her well, because this would be giving her too much power, which was the last thing his programming would allow.

As Bill continued to look deeply into his mind, he discovered quite a few more characteristics that caused him to manipulate people to his advantage in order to avoid his feeling of insignificance. The more aware he became of his negative programming, the more his compulsive need for attention from other people began to diminish. He saw clearly what his programming had turned him into, and he was determined to change.

After he had risen above his Jeffrey programming, Bill began dating a girl who was not the prettiest or most popular girl he could find, but instead, someone around whom he felt comfortable. With his new-found confidence, Bill was able to treat his new girlfriend much better than he had ever treated Claudia, because he was not intimidated by her. Claudia also met someone new, and she now receives the kindness, love, and appreciation she deserves.

Witnessing: A Path to Overcome
Family Disharmony

Angelo was a very sensitive child, born to a father who was stern, angry, and critical. The more sensitivity Angelo displayed, such as crying or needing to express himself, the more critical his father George would become. This led to a stormy relationship, which increased in its intensity with each passing year.

When Angelo graduated from high school, his mother landed in the hospital after having a heart attack. A Clergy was called in, and Angelo's mother shared that the disharmony between Angelo and George was too much for her to bear. Now that Angelo was moving out of the house, she feared that her husband and son would grow further apart and be at odds with each other forever. The Clergy recommended The Witnessing Technique to the family, so Angelo made an appointment right away.

The most painful feeling that Angelo experienced with his father was the feeling of being disconnected. He was invited to allow his feelings to form into an image, and the vision of a very high, thick, stone wall appeared. Angelo described it as looking like *The Great Wall of China*, a dreadful rock wall that seemed permanent and impenetrable. Angelo was encouraged to continue to observe the wall, recognizing that it only represented his fear, but that he could rise above his programming and change his reality if he wanted to do so.

When we continue to see things as they have always been, it is unlikely there will be any transformation. Opening to a more joyful reality, even if we do not know how to bring a new reality about, will lift us above the old programming, so that we can step into a new, improved experience quickly. Angelo understood that even if the wall appeared to be real in his life, he could find his own freedom from it, by dissolving his attachment to his fear.

Angelo returned one week later, excited to share that he no longer took his *Great Wall of China* programming personally. After five days of *witnessing* the image, he actually felt consistently neutral about the wall and was able to see the absurdity of its formation. From the *Witnessing* perspective, Angelo realized that the wall was not giving him a solution to his pain. In fact, it was making his desire for a connection with his father appear hopeless. Because the programming was beginning to lose its power over Angelo's perception of his relationship with George, he felt more open to the love he had once known for his father.

Angelo applied the technique in the presence of his father during a family get-together the following weekend, and his father did not have any blow-outs toward him, which was a first. This made Angelo feel more in control of his life, and he viewed it as quite a victory over his victim programming. He had finally found a way to remain powerful around George.

The next program Angelo wanted to work on overcoming was the hopelessness he felt in his pursuit to please or impress his father. He was guided to close his eyes and allow his hopelessness to form into an image, and the vision of a chicken appeared. Angelo described it as brainless, and shared that his father had often told his mother to throw Angelo out with the other brainless chickens in the backyard. In his mind, he began to regard himself with the same respect his father gave to the chickens, which was none at all.

The solution to this painful feeling, according to his ego, was to find a way to impress his father so that George would validate his existence for him. As the *witness,* however, Angelo already felt validated. He did not have to rely on his father's acceptance in order to feel good about himself.

During the next family get-together George was ill, and Angelo was called to his bedside. Angelo's father did not say anything to him when he entered, but he looked him in the eyes and smiled. Angelo was delighted and smiled back. They sat together silently for over half an hour until George fell sleep. This was the first time Angelo had ever experienced his father's acceptance. *There was nothing blocking Angelo's view anymore. His wall had come down.*

Angelo continues to practice The Witnessing Technique, and he is on close terms with his father now. They are two new people interacting with love and respect. It was only their inner fears which caused them to shut down to one another in the past. *As in Angelo's case, it often takes only one person in a situation to seek healing for a shift to occur in the relationship or within a family unit.*

Witnessing: A Path to Overcome

Programming with Love

True love in a partnership not only allows the programming in the mind to surface, but also inspires a commitment to rise above the ego, instead of choosing to discard the current lover in order to move on to the next person. When we love someone deeply, we are willing to transform into a less programmed person, even if it hurts the ego to do so.

Tory and Demi had been married for three years. Tory's personality was formed in defense of others perceiving him as bad or deviant. He tried to counteract this fear by following all the right rules, which in his mind would cause him to appear saint-like and orderly. Tory kept a spotless house, he carried his holy book with him wherever he went, and he visited his place of worship regularly. All of these behaviors made him feel safe, because he believed he would appear good in other people's eyes. However, he was more passionate about ironing his clothes than he was about spending time with his wife Demi.

Demi had been programmed to believe that she was unwanted and unworthy of love, which caused a desperate desire for constant affection and sexual attention. However, when Demi flaunted herself sexually in front of her husband, his programming deemed her behavior as bad, devious, or indulgent.

Tory felt justified in punishing Demi for her "deviance" by rejecting her harshly. According to Tory's programming, if he remained disciplined in the midst of sexual temptations, he would be seen as even more saint-like. If he was saint-like, he was sure Demi would have more reverence for him. Instead, Tory's behavior brought up Demi's programmed fears of being unworthy of love and unwanted. In defense of these fears, Demi's programming validated her desire to reach out to other men for love and attention, which led to a number of affairs.

Tory and Demi came in for a Witnessing session as a last attempt to understand one another and stay together. Just as most couples do, Tory and Demi were blaming one another for their anguish. Consequently, they were individually guided to uncover their own programming in turn. Demi was asked to express what feelings led to her affairs, and she shared that Tory did not have the time of day for her. When she wanted to make love, he wanted to read the Bible. When affection came easily and abundantly from other men, Demi had no ability to say no, because her programming made her feel starved for it.

Demi allowed her feelings of desperately needing sexual affection to form into an image, and the vision of a shattered ceramic heart appeared. The heart needed love, which she interpreted as sexual attention, to glue it back together. However, the image symbolized that no matter how much attention she received, she would never truly feel loved or wanted.

Demi was guided to become aware of the aspect of her consciousness that was able to observe the shattered ceramic heart. Once she had aligned with her *Witnessing Self,* she understood that it was only a belief in her mind that caused her to view herself as unwanted and unworthy of love.

As she continued to identify more with her *Witnessing Self,* her overly seductive behavior subsided, and Tory felt more comfortable responding to her. *Demi did not suppress any of her sexual feelings. They simply began to emerge in more subtle ways now that the energy was inspired by her love for Tory, instead of her need for him to validate her.*

When Tory was asked to express the feelings which led him to condemn his wife for her sexual advances toward him, Tory shared that he thought she needed to learn discipline and morals, and that she should read the Holy Scriptures and go to their place of worship with him. If she did not do these things, he saw her as bad, because she was focused more on pleasures than on discipline, and he was not about to become seduced by her "evil ways."

Tory allowed the feeling of condemnation for his wife to turn into an image, and the vision of a drill sergeant with a baton appeared. The drill sergeant was trying to whip everything into shape. He preached restraint, and he controlled those who did not follow his rules or commands.

As Tory learned to rise above his programming and identify with his *Witnessing Self,* the fears which led him to push his wife away diminished, and he was able to see Demi for who she was, instead of perceiving her through his programmed idea of good, bad, right and wrong. He also applied The Witnessing Technique to the negative beliefs he held about sexuality and soon found that he was less inhibited in the bedroom and more capable of enjoying Demi's loving, sensuous ways. Eventually, he became the instigator of the sexual unions with his wife, which delighted Demi even more. Tory and Demi continue to practice The Witnessing Technique every time there is a challenge which appears insurmountable in their marriage. They always find programming at its roots and have been able to successfully work it through quite quickly.

CHAPTER 14

Superhero Images

Witnessing Positive Images

AS WE LOOK INSIDE AND OBSERVE THE SYMBOLISM IN THE MIND, we will discover angry images which kill and destroy things. Some are sad images, which pout, cry, remain hopeless, and wait for people to notice, love, or rescue them. Some are frightened images which attack others, hide, or pretend they are dead, for example. These archetypes represent the way our ego responds to stress.

When the ego experiences desire, appealing characters will appear which reflect our yearning for perfection. Often Superhero's, which hold amazing powers and appear flawless, will arise, indicating how extraordinary the ego expects us to be in order to feel safe and secure in this world.

When we invest in our programmed beliefs about self, we rely on ideas which are less magnificent than our true identity.

Even the most angelic images will not hold a candle to the deep invigorating experience of your *Witnessing Self*. For this reason, we must also detach from the positive images in order to connect with our original identity. As you suspend yourself from the programming in this way, you will discover your *true self* and begin to lead an enchanted life.

Witnessing

A Superhero Image

Cameron lived quite happily with his girlfriend Patricia for three years. When he turned forty-nine, however, he became obsessed with a college girl named Mindy, who sold muffins at a deli across from his office. Frustrated with his intense infatuation, Cameron confided in his brother, who suggested The Witnessing Technique; explaining that it may offer clarity concerning his situation.

When Cameron arrived for his session, his face lit up while he described how beautiful, innocent, young, and voluptuous Mindy was. She appeared to be the perfect woman and the answer to his dreams. When the conversation shifted to his three year relationship with Patricia, all vitality in his face disappeared. He slumped over in his chair and covered his mouth with his hands, afraid of saying the wrong thing. He struggled to find things that excited him about Patricia, then eventually shared that he did not want to hurt her or break up with her.

The most intense emotion Cameron felt about his situation was the feeling of being trapped. He was guided to allow his feelings to form into an image, and the vision of a man behind bars appeared. The image glared out at his freedom with pathetic longing. Cameron was invited to become aware of the aspect of his consciousness that was able to observe the image, and he experienced a tremendous sense of freedom almost instantly. This transformation caused him to realize that a shift in perspective might allow him to enjoy Patricia more, if he did not feel trapped by her.

Cameron was still excited about Mindy, so he spent another few minutes describing the joy he experienced whenever he spoke with her, admitting that it would be a big ego boost to have such a beautiful girl to take to parties and other social events. When he was invited to allow his joy to form into an image, the vision of Superman appeared holding a dozen roses. Cameron was delighted with the image, stating that the vision made him feel better about himself than he ever remembered.

Cameron watched the character for a while, but eventually he became bored with Superman's flexing muscles and ulta-bright smile. Once he felt neutral, he was able to detach from the image, and identify with his *Witnessing Self*. Although Cameron believed that his superhero was the ultimate archetype, he was astonished to find that he felt even more powerful as the *witness*. His *Witnessing Self* not only felt more potent, it also had no attachment to possessing Mindy; which made him feel oddly relaxed.

As Cameron continued to practice The Witnessing Technique, he discovered programming that caused him to need something or someone that he could use in order to dazzle others and avoid being seen as ordinary. He wanted to be captivating and magical in other people's eyes. Now that he was getting older, he felt less appealing and his programming urged him to seek someone else who could make up for his growing insecurities. *This is the well-known mid-life crisis. As we age, our programming becomes more desperate and pressures us to improve our image with impressive outside additions.*

As Cameron continued to *witness* the insecurities in his mind, he eventually realized that he wanted to use Mindy. He never considered what she might want or what was important to her. As he spent more time chatting with her at the muffin shop, it became apparent they had nothing at all in common. Mindy wanted to marry a billionaire and have six children. Not only did Cameron not want to get married, he certainly did not want children. Once Cameron thought about honoring Mindy, all of his joy and excitement dissipated. It felt like too much work. His excitement had been about what he could *get* from her. *This is a very common recognition most people come across as they observe their ego.*

As Cameron continued to *witness* his Superman image, he was able to establish a connection with Pure Consciousness, which caused him to feel youthful, excited, and confident all on his own. He also became less attached to needing Patricia in his life for safety and more capable of ending his relationship with her in a kind manner. Once he did so, a new and more appropriate relationship entered his life.

~~~

CHAPTER 15

Well-Being

Witnessing

A Path to Total Well-Being

ALTHOUGH AN ENTIRE BOOK could have been written on any one of the important topics covered so far, this publishing was intended to introduce The Witnessing Technique so that readers could become acquainted with the astounding transformation anyone can experience with its application.

In addition to the topics covered so far, this technique has been successfully applied to transform health conditions, financial predicaments, career dilemmas, stage fright, writers block, fear of intimacy, sexual deviance, power struggles, impatience, disappointment, envy, hatred, guilt, trauma, regret, and lack of awareness.

The following examples demonstrate how mental programming can affect our well-being, and how simple it is to transform and improve any condition once we rise above the chaos in the mind and re-connect with our *Witnessing Self.*

Witnessing: A Path to Allow
Physical and Emotional Well-Being

Shanti devoted her life to protecting natural habitats by educating people on the delicacy and balance of the wilderness. When she turned thirty, she met a man who loved the outdoors as much as she did and had just as much thirst for adventure. Within a few months of dating Gil, however, she began having horrific asthma attacks, and she made an appointment to discover the root cause of her illness.

When Shanti called for her session, she shared that she had been under a lot of stress and that her boyfriend Gil was turning out to be quite a disappointment. She had also been experiencing a multitude of what she called, "ignorant people," who enraged her with their lack of respect for the well-being of animals and their environment.

When Shanti was directed to allow her feelings to form into an image, the vision of a Captain in charge of a large ship appeared. He had a lot of responsibilities and carried a burdening load on his shoulders. The Captain patrolled the deck of his ship, making sure everyone did everything *right*. If his crew proved to be incompetent, he felt it was all his fault. He took his job very seriously and had no tolerance for mistakes committed by himself or others.

The Captain portrayed a program in Shanti's mind that caused her to feel personally responsible for everyone else's actions. If she could not get her message across, she would condemn herself as a failure and feel a deep loathing for the incompetent people who had let her down. Every time she failed, her mind would jump to the conclusion that something was wrong with her. She was just not good enough, not smart enough, not wise enough, not respected enough, and not powerful enough. The more her mind focused on not being enough, the more frustrated she became.

Shanti was guided to allow her frustration to form into an image, and the vision of a red she-devil appeared. The devil was dressed in bright red leotards, and she spit fire at everyone who did not love and respect her, acknowledge how hard she was trying, or support her emotionally. When Shanti's boyfriend did anything that made her feel disrespected or unloved, her she-devil programming would take over and force her to throw verbal flames of anger at Gil. Her intent was to hurt him, make him wrong, and punish him as much as possible. Her rage consumed her and pushed her boyfriend away, working against her in the love arena.

Shanti was guided to identify with the aspect of her consciousness that was able to observe the image, and she immediately took a breath and relaxed. As the *witness,* she felt love flowing toward her, so she no longer had to rely on love from the outside world to feel safe. Once Shanti felt respected, acknowledged, and powerful from within, she had no reason to try to hurt others. In fact, when she was flowing with Pure Consciousness, she wanted others to feel loved as well.

Once she had worked through enough of her surface pain, she was asked to express the most intense event that had occurred right before she'd had her first asthma attack. Shanti suddenly became enraged and began sharing what her boyfriend had done, how stupid some of the people around her were, and how much harm men were causing the planet. She felt helpless to change the world immediately, which was what she expected she should be able to do.

Shanti was guided to allow her feelings of exasperation to form into an image, and a vision of white vapor rising up into the atmosphere appeared.

The vapor was leaving the planet and moving out into space. Shanti shared that the vapor was her Life Force. *When she saw herself as a failure, her hopelessness made her choose to give up and get a head start on leaving, instead of continuing to try harder to prove that she was good enough, which seemed impossible.* According to Shanti's programming, the only reason for being alive was to make a difference and be of service on the planet, and she was determined to match the perfect idea of being selfless and of service that her mind had projected.

As the *witness*, however, she realized that her actions had nothing to do with her right to exist or her worth. Her peaceful *beingness*, experienced by identifying with her *Witnessing Self*, was of service to the planet in a more profound way than all of her rageful thoughts and actions toward the "bad" people could have ever been. Her programmed idea of *service* was, in fact, a *disservice* to herself and others. Shanti eventually recognized that the responsibility of the world was not on her shoulders. All she had to do to make a difference was connect with the peaceful, loving energy of Pure Consciousness and follow its gentle guidance.

Always wanting to do her best, Shanti has not had a recurrence of her asthma ever since she discovered the image of the white vapor. She has also experienced great success rising above her she-devil programming, and more love and positive acknowledgement are flowing her way.

Witnessing: A Path to Overcome

Accident-Prone Programming

Julie had been in five car accidents in two years, so a friend suggested she work with The Witnessing Technique to discover what might be causing these recurring events. When she arrived for her session, she appeared exceedingly business-like and stern. She had a list of everything she wanted to cover, and she went through it very methodically.

The first challenge she wanted to address concerned her boyfriend. In a huff, Julie shared that she had discovered him doing his laundry at 1:00 in the afternoon. The correct rules that had come over the radio were never to use any electrical appliance between the hours of 8:00 a.m. and 6:00 p.m. in order to conserve energy. Julie lifted her head quite high as she expressed how strictly she adhered to this rule.

When she was asked why she thought her boyfriend had done his laundry at 1:00 pm, she replied, "First of all, he is stupid. I found him doing his laundry, because it is the only break he has between classes, and his night job, and the only time we can see each other. But he should rearrange his schedule so he could do laundry at the proper time. How do you think it makes me look to have a boyfriend who does his laundry in the middle of the day?"

Julie was guided to close her eyes and sense what feelings arose when she came across people who were not following her rules. Her face turned crimson and her whole body stiffened. She shared that it was not fair that she had to be the only good person on earth and she wanted justice. Julie was invited to allow her emotions to form into an image, and the vision of a very authoritative looking Judge appeared in her mind. His court room hammer was held up high, ready to condemn those to whom he felt superior.

When Julie was guided to identify with the aspect of her consciousness that was able to observe the image, she blurted out that every motorist she had cut off deserved her punishment, because they had to be made aware of their actions. Julie was asked if it was worth risking her life to show people when they had made a mistake, and she quickly replied, "God will protect me. I am on his side."

In Julie's most recent accident, however, she had refused to let another motorist enter the freeway from an on-ramp. When room ran out in her lane, she stepped on the gas and hit him on his left side as hard as she could, intending to show the other motorist that he was at fault. The investigating police officer found it to be Julie's fault, however, because she had failed to allow the merging traffic to enter the freeway. She also suffered severe foot lacerations when the entire front end of her vehicle was crushed.

Julie was asked to review this most recent accident to decide if she had been suspended from any repercussions, or if it appeared that she sustained more damage than the person she had intended to punish. Never having considered these factors before, she agreed to think about it throughout the week.

When Julie arrived for her next session she was very upset. Her boyfriend had broken up with her, because she was too judgmental and always found fault with him no matter what he did. She told him that if he did not have so many faults, she would not have to bring them up. Before Julie left him, she looked him in the eyes and told him he was a bad person.

His response was, "You are wrong about that." That had incensed her. She was guided to allow her feelings of being thought of as "wrong" to form into an image, and the vision of a man with devil horns appeared. Condemned by the church, his head had been locked into a guillotine, preparing him for execution. The man felt shame and humiliation for his sins, but he was unable to do anything about it. The image wanted to prove himself to be innocent and be redeemed in front of the whole world.

Julie was very disturbed by the image and shared that it reminded her of her grandmother, who was very religious. When Julie was a child, her grandmother would tell her to watch out for the devil inside of herself, warning that it would force her to do bad things. Julie had been watchful ever since and quick to point out to others when she had done the *right* thing or performed a good deed. She wanted to make it perfectly clear that she did not have the devil inside of herself.

When Julie was guided to connect with the aspect of her consciousness that was able to observe the image, she felt immediately detached from her fear of being bad and wrong; which gave her a whole new perspective on life. As time went on, she became aware of why she acted the way she did on the road and how severe and unnecessary her previous actions had been.

Julie eventually realized that even as a small child in front of her grandmother, she had always been innocent, and there had never been anything to prove. Once she had risen above her programming, she no longer experienced road rage, and her relationships with others became much more harmonious.

Witnessing: A Path to Overcome

Lack Consciousness

As an investment broker, Stephen's life revolved around his own money and the finances of others. When Stephen's bills arrived, he would hold off on paying everything until the last minute, so that he could enjoy his abundant bank balance and feel proud. When he owed money to someone who was not part of a large corporation, he had no intention of paying them at all. He knew that in order for them to collect their money from him, it would cost them more in legal fees for it to be worth their while. Stephen thought this was quite a smart move financially. He liked the idea of creditors calling him, because in his mind, he had their money and they had to beg for it.

Stephen resented having to pay for anything, and he refused to purchase health insurance, seeing no reason to have it while he was in perfect health. In his mid-thirties, however, Stephen began having terrible pain in his abdomen. When he went in for a check up, the doctors discovered cancer had spread throughout his colon. Stephen reluctantly agreed to enter a facility which treated people without insurance, but he felt tremendous resentment over having to pay their fees.

After three months of chemotherapy, Stephen's condition had worsened, so he decided to sue the hospital for malpractice. His health diminished so rapidly, however, that he was unable to concentrate on anything but his pain. One day he was visited by a volunteer counselor who often spent time with cancer patients at the low rate facility. The counselor was shocked to see Stephen receiving discounted care, as he knew of his great wealth through adds in the local papers promoting his business. Noticing that Stephen was not responding to medical treatment, the counselor suggested The Witnessing Technique, so Stephen made an appointment that day.

When Stephen called for his session, he shared that terror was his most predominant emotion, so he was guided to allow his fear to form into an image, and the vision of a scrawny scarecrow with straw falling out of his tattered clothing appeared. Crows were lurking around, but the scarecrow had little effect, because he looked frightened himself. The scarecrow was in a field of golden hay which looked like gold coins, but the coins were weightless and they could float away on the breeze. *Stephen believed that if he could not frighten people or have power over them, his money would be taken away. It was easy to lose, so he always had to be the scarecrow making sure no one came into his field.*

When Stephen was guided to become aware of the aspect of his consciousness that was able to observe the image, he realized that he did not have to identify with the scarecrow programming and live in fear any longer. His *Witnessing Self* had no fear of lack or deprivation. As the *witness*, he was already fulfilled and stable in every way, so he had no concern over money. This was an awakening experience for Stephen, because he had always associated having money with having a lot of stress in order to keep it. Now he realized that having an abundance consciousness made having money fun. All he had to do was identify with his wise, aware *Witnessing Self*, and his money stress would evaporate.

Within two weeks of practicing the technique, Stephen's doctors announced that his body was starting to respond positively to the treatment. He was also delighted to discover his investments were earning more, and he was beginning to attract very affluent clientele with the kind of money he had always dreamed of investing. Now that his consciousness was focused more on abundance instead of the lack of it, he was attracting real wealth into his life.

Stephen diligently practices The Witnessing Technique each day in order to rise above his ego, and he continues to find greater delight, better health, and a positive attitude toward life and prosperity.

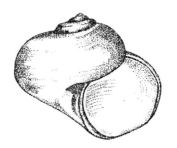

Conclusion

Insanity

THE LOWEST STATE OF THE HUMAN CONDITION IS INSANITY. Insanity occurs when thoughts, beliefs, and emotions dictate behavior to such an extent that an individual no longer has the ability to control his own mind, similar to a computer commanding its owner. Unfortunately, the masses operate with only a slightly higher degree of control over the mind than the clinically insane.

Our thoughts, beliefs, and feelings create our reality and attract to us our experiences. Therefore, it is of the utmost importance that we take back control from the mind and learn to wield our thoughts and emotions in the direction of our greater good. When we rise above the mind by connecting with our *Witnessing Self,* we gain authority over all of our energies, which gives us the power to create anything we want.

Once we rise above the mind,
the drama and insanity of life
will appear to be a movie we once watched.

In a movie theater, we agree to become identified with the images on the screen, living vicariously through the actors for a period of time. When the lights come on, however, we re-emerge into our own reality, realizing that the images on the screen were merely a projection. The mind itself is a non-stop movie. We agree to identify with the thoughts and emotions it projects and live vicariously through its drama, until we re-emerge into a higher reality and free ourselves from the conflict and trauma it contains. Those who identify with the mind's images exclusively, eventually lose their sanity.

We have the choice to be controlled by the mind and its negative patterns, or we can be guided by the freedom of our *Witnessing Self.* As the *witness,* you begin to realize that you are not the thoughts, feelings, or beliefs in the mind. You are not even this body. Your awareness *observes* all of these things, and this awareness or *Witnessing Self,* is the true you. You are Pure Consciousness, a wise, uplifting, creative power with authority over all conditions in life.

Enlightenment

The highest level of human potential or human consciousness is known as Enlightenment. The Enlightened Master has risen above the attachments of his ego in order to align with Source Energy. Light, clarity, and universal truth illuminate one's consciousness in this state.

While the mind is in control, we can at most access ten percent of our brain. The remaining ninety percent needs the elixir of Pure Consciousness to awaken it safely. This ninety percent is the key to our evolution. Without it, we see mankind falling to further depths of destruction.

Great geniuses, such as Pythagoras, Socrates, Epicurus, Bodhidharma, Goethe, Moses, Jesus, Gurdjieff, Lao Tzu and Rajneesh, were men who were masters of their own minds. They had tremendous awareness and great understanding of Pure Consciousness, which opened the doors to insights and discoveries far surpassing anything else available during their time. It is because of these people, and those of their caliber, that our world has evolved at all.

A deep connection with Pure Consciousness is the base for all higher knowing. We must reach beyond the mind to ignite our true potential and live free from the pain and illusions generated by the ego.

Beyond Enlightenment

Once a state of illumination has been reached, identification with male or female, black or white, Asian or Indian, Buddhist or Christian, Mohammedan or Hindu, Atheist or Theist, Marxist or Capitalist, Republican or Democrat, rich or poor, happy or sad, good or bad, etc., dissolves. The Enlightened one perceives his "being" as pure energy, flowing through life with no agenda, no attachments, no limitations, and no judgments. This pure, free energy is *bliss*.

*The path toward bliss can be found
in having mastery over the mind.*

Once you have mastered your mind, an aura of power and beauty will surround you. Your inner silence will touch people as they pass, uplifting them as if you were the sunrise itself. Simply move through life with greater awareness each day, and this blissfulness will begin to permeate your being, lifting you to heights beyond this world of ego and pain.

Your *Witnessing Self* is something you *can* and *will* take with you when you die, unlike your mind, your belongings, your title, status or partner. It is a connection with your eternal source, and it is the most essential treasure in which you can invest. As the *witness,* you are diving into the mysteries of Existence—reaching beyond where most people ever dream of living—and merging with the miraculous.

About the Author and the Techniques

During her in-depth study of *consciousness*, Miss Bisset noticed that the ability to rise above the drama of the mind by *observing reality*, instead of *personalizing it*, reaped the most profound transformation in consciousness and the greatest understanding of *self*. Intending to offer this insight to others, Miss Bisset developed two techniques which she has coined:

"The Witnessing Technique and The Love Meditation"

These techniques offer a simple and straightforward approach to rise above the mind and view all drama and pain from an impartial perspective. From this place, one learns to *identify* with an aspect of consciousness that is free from the mind's limiting programming, allowing an ecstatic taste of Pure Consciousness to be experienced.

Because these techniques are performed regularly, transformation is swift. Inner conflicts and limiting thoughts rapidly disappear and create an opening for greater clarity, power, and joy. By mastering the mind, we access our true potential and discover the secret to wielding our power— which makes us all Divine.

Addictions, obsessions, compulsions, neurosis, and traumas are rooted in the mind. Therefore, any dysfunction or painful occurrence dissolves as an individual learns to identify with a higher, more intelligent, and evolved aspect of one's *being*, hence the effectiveness of these techniques.